NPTE
CHEAT SHEETS

LEARN THE TOUGHEST NPTE CONCEPTS IN
5 MINUTES OR LESS

Dr. Kyle Rice, PT, OCS

TABLE OF CONTENTS

SECTION 1 **MUSCULOSKELETAL CHEAT SHEETS** 1

CHAPTER 1	AFO TYPES & FUNCTIONS	3
CHAPTER 2	ASSISTIVE DEVICES	7
CHAPTER 3	CLINICAL PREDICTION RULES	13
CHAPTER 4	CONGENITAL MUSCULAR TORTICOLLIS	19
CHAPTER 5	END FEELS	23
CHAPTER 6	FEMALE ATHLETE TRIAD	29
CHAPTER 7	FEMORAL TORSION	33
CHAPTER 8	FOOT MECHANICS	39
CHAPTER 9	GAIT DEVIATIONS	45
CHAPTER 10	GOUT	51
CHAPTER 11	HISTORY TAKING	57
CHAPTER 12	INNOMINATE ROTATIONs	63
CHAPTER 13	ISOKINETIC TESTING	67
CHAPTER 14	LUMBAR MECHANICAL TRACTION	71
CHAPTER 15	MEDIAL MENISCAL TEAR	75
CHAPTER 16	MSK BREATHING MECHANICS	79
CHAPTER 17	MUSCULOSKELETAL DIAGNOSTIC IMAGING	85
CHAPTER 18	PLUMB LINE	91
CHAPTER 19	PROSTHETIC GAIT DEVIATIONS	95
CHAPTER 20	REVERSE MUSCLE ACTIONS	99
CHAPTER 21	RHEUMATOID & OSTEO ARTHRITIS	105
CHAPTER 22	SHIN PAIN	109
CHAPTER 23	SHOULDER SPECIAL TESTS	115
CHAPTER 24	SLAP TEAR ORTHOPEDIC PROTOCOL	121
CHAPTER 25	SLIPPED CAPITAL FEMORAL EPIPHYSIS	127

CHAPTER 26	SPONDYLOLISTHESIS	131
CHAPTER 27	THUMB MECHANICS	137
CHAPTER 28	TMJ BASICS	141
CHAPTER 29	TRICKY TRANSFERS	147
CHAPTER 30	VBI TESTING	151
CHAPTER 31	TYPES OF PAIN	157
CHAPTER 32	DISTINGUISHING PAIN	163
REFERENCES		167

SECTION II NEUROMUSCULAR CHEAT SHEETS ... 171

CHAPTER 33	APHASIA	173
CHAPTER 34	CENTRAL CORD SYNDROME DIFFERENTIAL	179
CHAPTER 35	COMMON FEEDBACK TYPES	183
CHAPTER 36	CRANIAL NERVES	189
CHAPTER 37	GROSS MOTOR FUNCTION AND CEREBRAL PALSY	193
CHAPTER 38	LATERAL MEDULLARY SYNDROME	197
CHAPTER 39	MYASTHENIA GRAVIS	201
CHAPTER 40	NEURAL TENSION TESTING	207
CHAPTER 41	PARKINSONIAN GAIT INTERVENTIONS	211
CHAPTER 42	PNF LEAD ARM	217
CHAPTER 43	PUSHER'S SYNDROME	223
CHAPTER 44	SPINA BIFIDA	229
CHAPTER 45	STAGES OF MOTOR LEARNING	231
CHAPTER 46	TRAUMATIC BRAIN INJURY	235
CHAPTER 47	VESTIBULAR SPECIAL TESTING	241
CHAPTER 48	VESTIBULAR REHAB	247
REFERENCES		251

SECTION III CARDIOPULMONARY CHEAT SHEETS 253

CHAPTER 49	6-MINUTE WALK TEST	255
CHAPTER 50	ALTITUDE & CARDIOPULMONARY	261
CHAPTER 51	AQUATIC THERAPY	265
CHAPTER 52	ARTERIAL INSUFFICIENCY	269
CHAPTER 53	BLOOD GASES	273
CHAPTER 54	EKG INTERPRETATION	279
CHAPTER 55	EXERCISE RESPONSES	287
CHAPTER 56	HEART SOUNDS	293
CHAPTER 57	HEMODIALYSIS	299
CHAPTER 58	LAB VALUES	303
CHAPTER 59	NPTE BIOMARKERS	307
CHAPTER 60	PNEUMONIA	313
CHAPTER 61	ACUTE CARE LINES	317
CHAPTER 62	PULMONARY MEDICATIONS	323
CHAPTER 63	PULMONARY INTERVENTIONS	329
CHAPTER 64	RESTRICTIVE AND OBSTRUCTIVE CONDITIONS	337
CHAPTER 65	EXERCISE INTENSITY MEASURES	341
CHAPTER 66	ABNORMAL BREATHING PATTERNS	345
REFERENCES		351

SECTION IV OTHER SYSTEMS 353

CHAPTER 67	TYPES OF ULCERS	355
CHAPTER 68	ABCDE METHOD OF MELANOMA	361
CHAPTER 69	LYMPHEDEMA VS LIPEDEMA	365
CHAPTER 70	BURNS	369
CHAPTER 71	DIABETES IMPLICATIONS	373
CHAPTER 72	PERSONAL PROTECTIVE EQUIPMENT	377

CHAPTER 73	PULSED LAVAGE		381
CHAPTER 74	TOP NAIL TYPES		385
CHAPTER 75	CUSHING'S AND ADDISON'S		391
CHAPTER 76	TOP 7 TOPICAL AGENTS6		397
CHAPTER 77	HYPOTHYROIDISM		403
CHAPTER 78	GENITOURINARY DIFFERENTIAL DIAGNOSIS		407
CHAPTER 79	VISCERAL PAIN PATTERNS		413
REFERENCES			417

SECTION V — NON-SYSTEMS CHEAT SHEETS — 419

CHAPTER 80	BEHAVIOR CHANGE		421
CHAPTER 81	INTERPRETING THE BELL CURVE		425
CHAPTER 82	COGNITIVE BEHAVIORAL THERAPY		431
CHAPTER 83	FUNCTIONAL ELECTRICAL STIMULATION		437
CHAPTER 84	PROSTHETIC K-LEVELS		443
CHAPTER 85	PT & PTA RESPONSIBILITIES		447
CHAPTER 86	STATISTICAL POWER		449
CHAPTER 87	TENS		453
CHAPTER 88	THE FLAG SYSTEM		459
CHAPTER 89	THERAPEUTIC ULTRASOUND		463
CHAPTER 90	TOP 10 NPTE MEDICATIONS HIT LIST		469
CHAPTER 91	TOP 10 NPTE OUTCOME MEASURES		471
CHAPTER 92	WHEELCHAIRS, RAMPS & ADA GUIDELINES		475
CHAPTER 93	NPTE ABBREVIATIONS & ACRONYMS		479
REFERENCES			483

ABOUT THE AUTHOR 484
ACKNOWLEDGEMENTS 485

DISCLAIMER:

The information provided in these cheat sheets is to help answer questions on the National Physical Therapy Examination. By no means is the information in this book to be used as specific recommendations for any patient(s) being treated in the clinic or hospital. Since each clinical situation/presentation can be different, clinical judgment should be exercised.

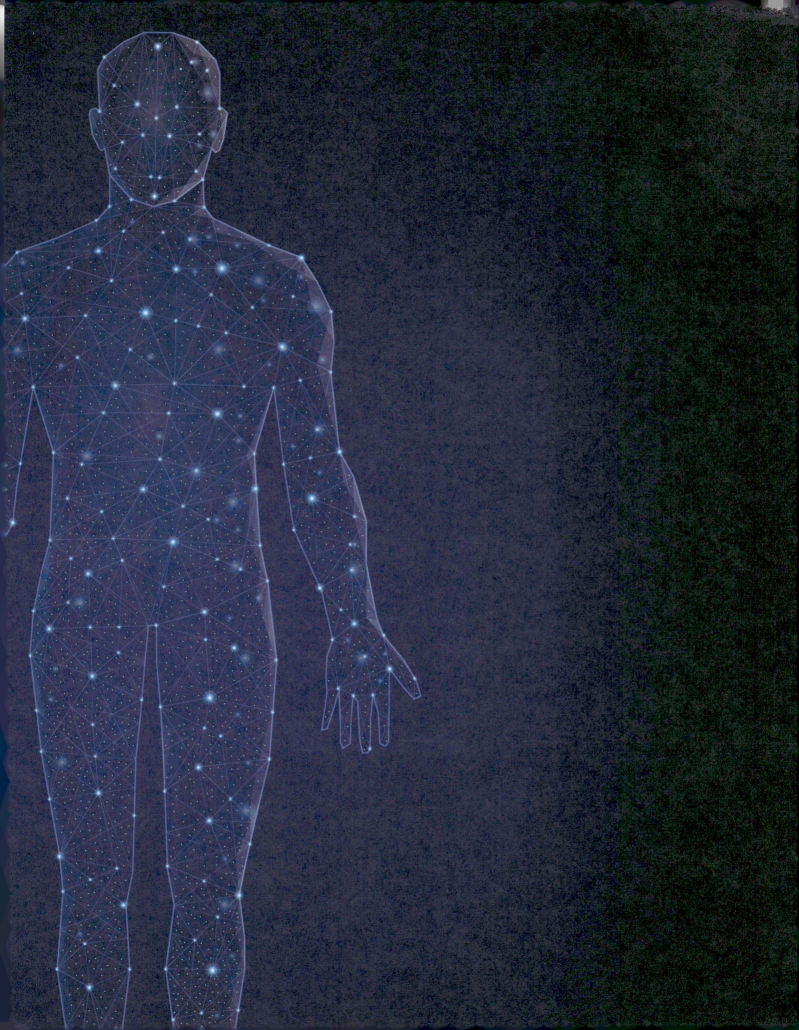

SECTION I

MUSCULOSKELETAL CHEAT SHEETS

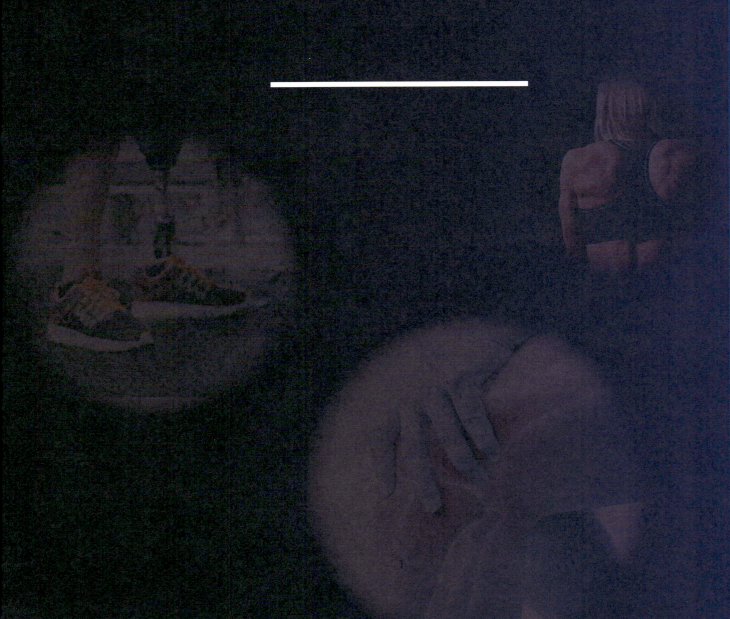

CHAPTER 1

AFO TYPES & FUNCTIONS

SECTION I

TOP 3 AFO TYPES & FUNCTIONS

ARTICULATED (HINGED) ANKLE FOOT ORTHOSIS[1]

Basic construction:

Hybrid, hinged, or articulated AFOs comprise a calf component that is separate from but articulates with a footplate.

Why are Articulated AFOs often selected?

To allow free unrestricted sagittal plane motion at the ankle while limiting medial/lateral ankle motion.

Modifications added to these AFOs:

1. Posterior Stop
    a. A buttress on the rear aspect of the AFO that stops excessive plantarflexion.

2. Dorsiflexion Stop
    a. Typically, a Velcro strap on the posterior aspect of the AFO that limits excessive dorsiflexion.

When are these AFOs often prescribed?

1. If a Solid AFO (SAFO) provides too much rigidity beyond the patient's needs.

2. Patients who require medial/lateral stability at the ankle but are active. (Negotiate stairs, ramps, curbs, etc.)

3. Patients with spastic cerebral palsy, knee hyperextension, and/or correctable ankle equinus.

CHAPTER 1

POSTERIOR LEAF SPRING AFO[2]

Basic construction:
Flexible co-polymer polypropylene or carbon fiber that typically allows for stored energy potential.

Why are PLS-AFOs often selected?
To assist with ankle dorsiflexion and foot clearance during the swing phase.

When are these AFOs often prescribed?
1. If a patient has mild spastic cerebral palsy or a condition producing isolated dorsiflexor weakness or paralysis.

2. If a patient requires little to no medial/lateral ankle support.

3. If a patient needs minimal restriction of sagittal plane ankle motion.

GROUND REACTION ANKLE FOOT ORTHOSIS (GRAFO)[3]

Basic construction:
The GRAFO consists of a solid plastic material with a solid ankle. The upper portion of the AFO wraps around the anterior part of the proximal tibia.

Why are GRAFOs often selected?
To allow for control of both the ankle and the knee. This AFO prevents the knee from collapsing into flexion during the stance phase by restricting dorsiflexion at the ankle.

When are these AFOs often prescribed?
1. Patients who have knee buckling during the stance phase or present with a crouched gait posturing.

2. Patients with SCI, CVA, Multiple Sclerosis, Guillan Barre, or other neurological conditions causing weakness of the quadriceps.

NOTE: *For the GRAFO to be effective, the patient should have at least a 3/5 MMT of the quadriceps and good hip stability.*

CHAPTER 2

ASSISTIVE DEVICES

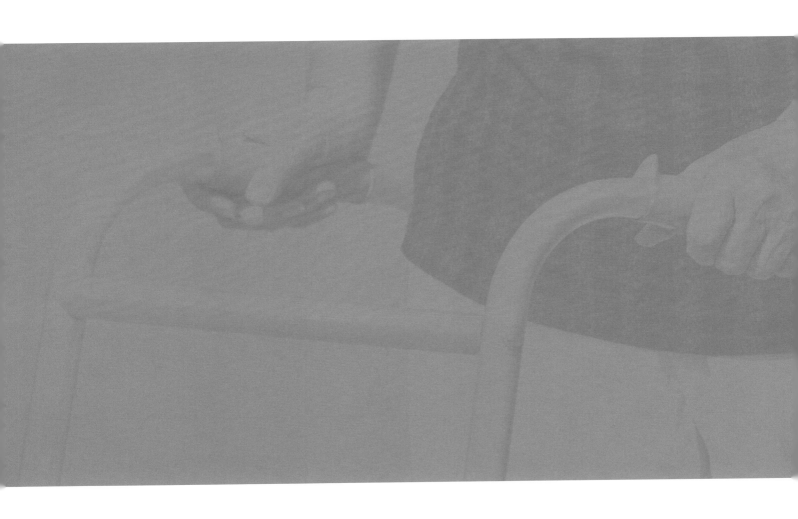

SECTION I

TOP 4 ASSISTIVE DEVICES[4]

STANDARD STRAIGHT CANE

Canes are used to compensate for impaired balance and to improve stability. Although the cane assists with balance, compared to other devices, the cane provides minimal support.

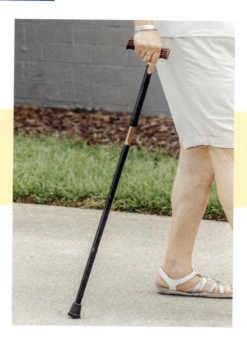

NPTE NOTES:
When selecting the appropriate cane height, the cane handle should be level with the patient's greater trochanter, ulnar styloid, or wrist crease.

Avoid the use of canes when the patient has lower extremity weight-bearing precautions.

LOFSTRAND (CANADIAN) CRUTCHES

Lofstrand crutches are used when the support and stability of axillary crutches are not needed but when the patient requires more support than a cane.

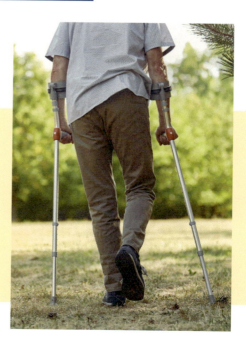

NPTE NOTES:
- The Lofstrand crutches **are often selected over axillary crutches when the patient has or is likely to have an injury to the axillary nerves and blood vessels.**
- Lofstrand crutches are **less stable than axillary crutches** and require functional standing balance and functional upper extremity strength.
- Lofstrand crutches are **infrequently used with elderly patients** because these patients feel insecure using them.

CHAPTER 2

AXILLARY CRUTCHES

Axillary crutches are provided when the patient needs less stability or support than is provided by a walker or parallel bars. These crutches allow faster speeds, various gait patterns, and better maneuverability.

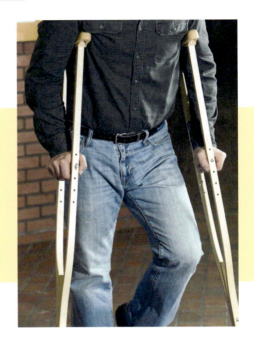

NPTE NOTES:
- Typically, axillary crutches are for **younger patients with functional upper extremities and adequate trunk strength.**
- Patients **require good standing balance when using axillary crutches.**
- These crutches **can cause injury to the axillary region**, including the nerves and blood vessels.

STANDARD WALKER

Typically, walkers are for patients who require maximal stability and support. These assistive devices are considered the most restrictive. Often, elderly patients or young children with neurological pathologies will use walkers.

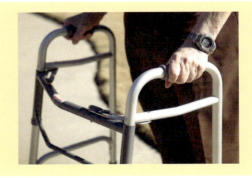

NPTE NOTES:
- Patients with a significant fall risk, lack of coordination, and/or impaired stability should use walkers.
- Walkers are the most restrictive device. Therefore, other less restrictive options that provide patient safety should be exhausted first.
- Walkers can be challenging to manage on stairs or in tight, confined spaces.

"TODAY'S PERFORMANCE DOESN'T DETERMINE WHAT YOU'RE CAPABLE OF ACHIEVING."

–COACH K

CHAPTER 3

CLINICAL PREDICTION RULES

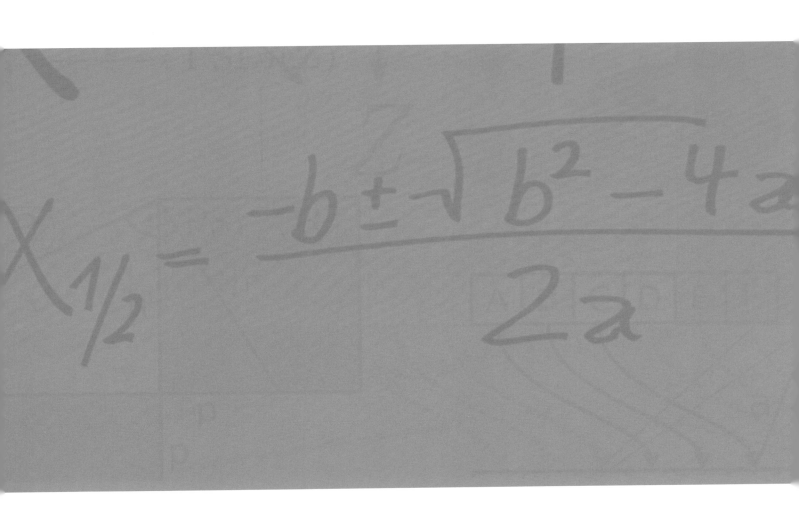

SECTION I

WHAT ARE CLINICAL PREDICTION RULES (CPRS)?

Mathematical tools intended to guide physiotherapists in their everyday clinical decision-making. CPRs act as evidence-based tools that physical therapists can use to diagnose, determine patient prognosis, and/or provide treatments that have the greatest likelihood of success. Rigorously tested and validated, most CPRs offer invaluable information to the clinician.

CERVICAL RADICULOPATHY CPR[5]

Cervical radiculopathy is highly likely (+ Likelihood Ratio: 30.3) to be present if all four characteristics are present:
- Positive upper limb tension test A (ULTTa)
- Involved-side cervical rotation range of motion less than 60 degrees.
- Positive Distraction test
- Positive Spurling's test A

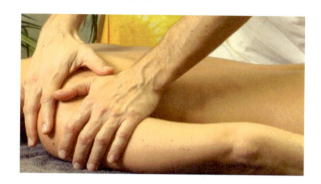

CARPAL TUNNEL CPR[6]

Carpal Tunnel Syndrome is likely (+ Likelihood Ratio: 4.3) to be present if at least 4 out of 5 characteristics are present:
- Shaking hands to relieve symptoms.
- Wrist ratio >.67
- Symptom Severity Scale > 1.9
- Diminished sensation in median sensory field 1 (thumb)
- Age > 45 years old

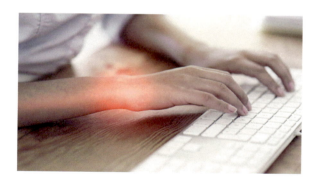

LUMBAR MANIPULATION CPR[7]

Considered/performed if at least four out of five characteristics are present:
- Pain lasts less than 16 days.
- No symptoms distal to the knee
- FABQ score less than 19.
- Internal rotation of greater than 35 degrees for at least one hip
- Hypomobility of at least one level of the lumbar spine

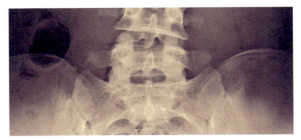

OTTAWA ANKLE RULES CPR[8]

An ankle x-ray is only required if there is pain present in the malleolar zone AND ANY ONE of the following are present:
- Bone tenderness along the distal 6 cm of the posterior edge of the tibia or tip of the medial malleolus

OR
- Bone tenderness along the distal 6 cm of the posterior edge of the fibula or tip of the lateral malleolus

OR
- An inability to bear weight immediately and in the emergency department for four steps.

OTTAWA FOOT RULES CPR[9]

A foot x-ray is only required if there is pain present in the midfoot zone AND ANY ONE of the following are present:
- Bone tenderness at the base of the fifth metatarsal (for foot injuries)

OR
- Bone tenderness at the navicular bone (for foot injuries)

OR
- An inability to bear weight both immediately and in the emergency department for four steps

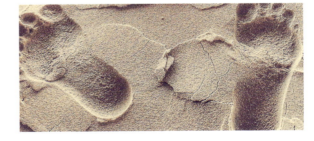

"PROBLEMS IN LIFE ARE INEVITABLE... LIFE IS JUST A GAME OF CHOOSING WHICH TYPE OF PROBLEMS YOU WANT"

–COACH K

CHAPTER 4

CONGENITAL MUSCULAR TORTICOLLIS

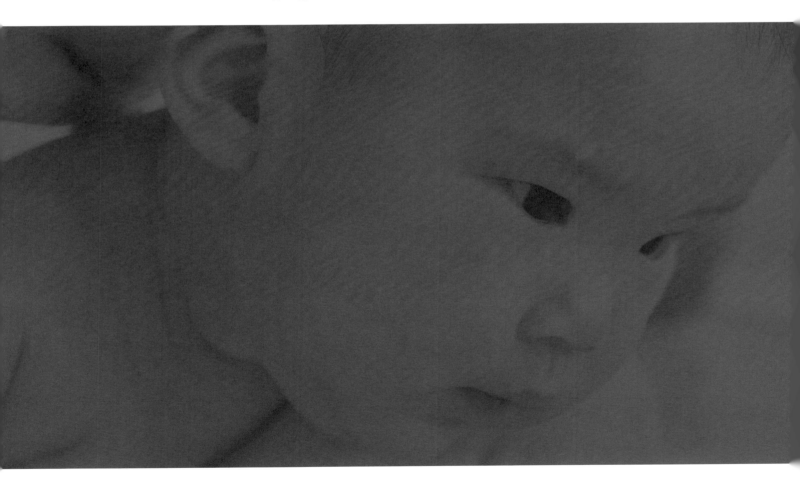

SECTION I

TORTICOLLIS

STERNOCLEIDOMASTOID (SCM)

This muscle connects to the sternum, clavicle, and mastoid process of the temporal bone. It *performs ipsilateral cervical side-bending and contralateral cervical rotation*.

CONGENITAL MUSCULAR TORTICOLLIS (CMT)

Also known as torticollis, it results from *unilateral shortening of the sternocleidomastoid (SCM) muscle. Often named for the side of the involved SCM muscle*.

DEFORMATIONAL PLAGIOCEPHALY (DP)[10]

In children, DP is a common condition that occurs in conjunction with torticollis. Typically, children with CMT will present with contralateral flattening of the skull.

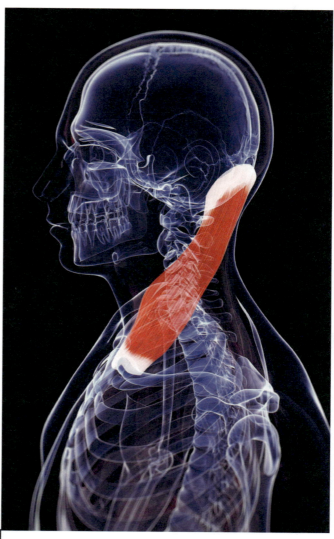

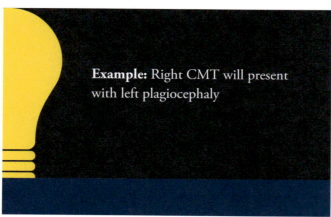

Example: Right CMT will present with left plagiocephaly

"WINNERS AREN'T THOSE WHO NEVER FAIL... IT'S THOSE WHO NEVER GIVE UP."

–COACH K

CHAPTER 5

END FEELS

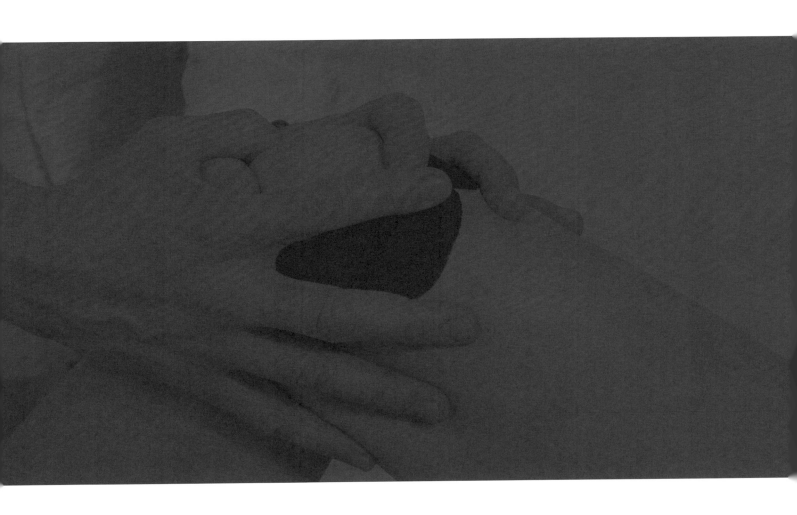

SECTION I

TYPES OF END FEELS[11,12]

- During a musculoskeletal examination, assessing passive motion is essential in determining the underlying condition.
- During passive range of motion testing, the physical therapist should apply overpressure at the end of ROM to determine the quality of the "end feel."
- The end feel is the sensation the examiner feels in the joint as it reaches the end of the range of motion.

NORMAL END FEELS	EXAMPLE
Bone to bone contact (Hard)	Elbow extension
Soft tissue approximation (Mushy Feel)	Elbow or knee flexion
Firm (Capsular)	Knee extension, MCP extension
Elastic-soft	Ankle Dorsiflexion

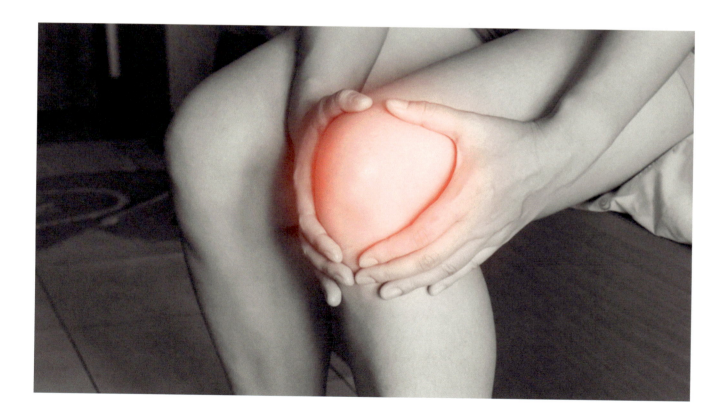

ABNORMAL END FEELS	QUALITY OF MOVEMENT	EXAMPLE
Capsular (Firm)	Thicker stretchy quality, no rebound	Frozen shoulder, TMJ capsular fibrosis
Soft Capsular (Boggy)	Normal tissue stretch and feel with a restricted range of motion	Swelling, Synovitis
Muscle Spasm	Sudden and hard arrest of movement often accompanied by pain	Cervical muscle spasms (cervical strain)
Springy Block	Rebound effect with a thick, stretchy feel	Meniscal tear, loose cartilage fragments in the joint
Empty	Movement stops because of the pain, although no natural mechanical resistance is detected	Pain, Acute subacromial bursitis, Tumor
Unexpected Bone to Bone	Sudden and hard stop before full range of motion	Osteophyte formation

"ANYTHING WORTH HAVING IS WORTH FAILING AT MULTIPLE TIMES."

–COACH K

CHAPTER 6

FEMALE ATHLETE TRIAD

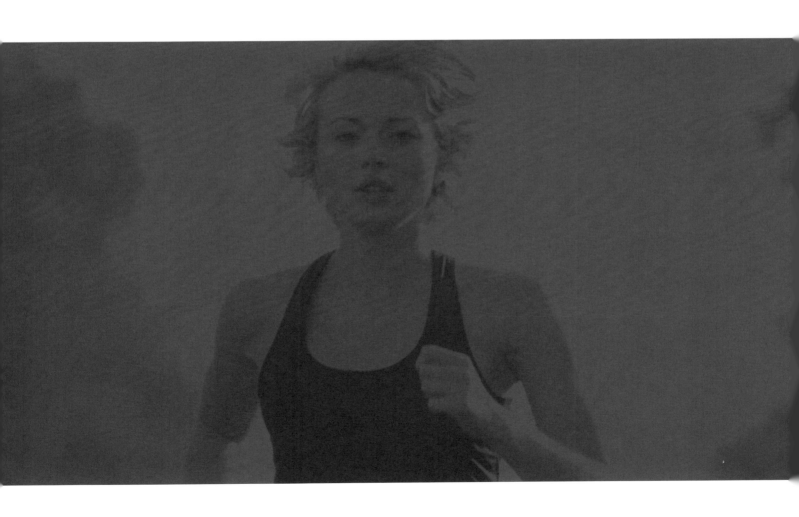

SECTION I

FEMALE TRIAD

The female athlete triad is a commonly underdiagnosed disorder composed of three interrelated conditions associated with athletic training:

E.O.A.[13]

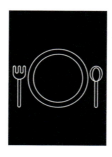

Eating Disorders
Female athletes with disordered eating may engage in several harmful eating behaviors to stave weight gain and maintain a thin physique.

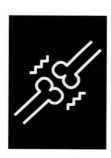

Osteoporosis
Estrogen, one of the significant hormones essential for bone health, is depleted in patients with female triad. This diminished bone density leads to recurrent stress fractures.

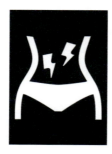

Amenorrhea
Amenorrhoea is the absence of menstrual periods. The most common cause is hormone disruption, which can be due to emotional stress, extreme weight loss, excessive exercise, or certain reproductive disorders. Changes in the Hypothalamus cause amenorrhea.

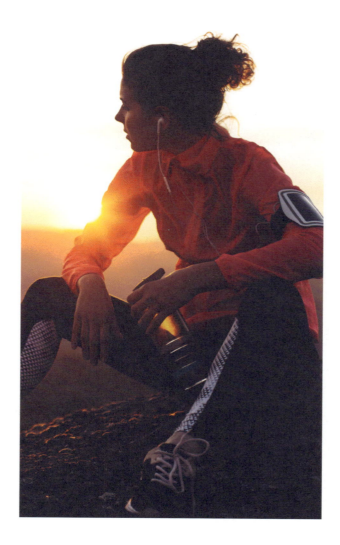

"IF IT'S NOT GOOD, GOD'S NOT DONE"

—TAUREN WELLS

CHAPTER 7

FEMORAL TORSION

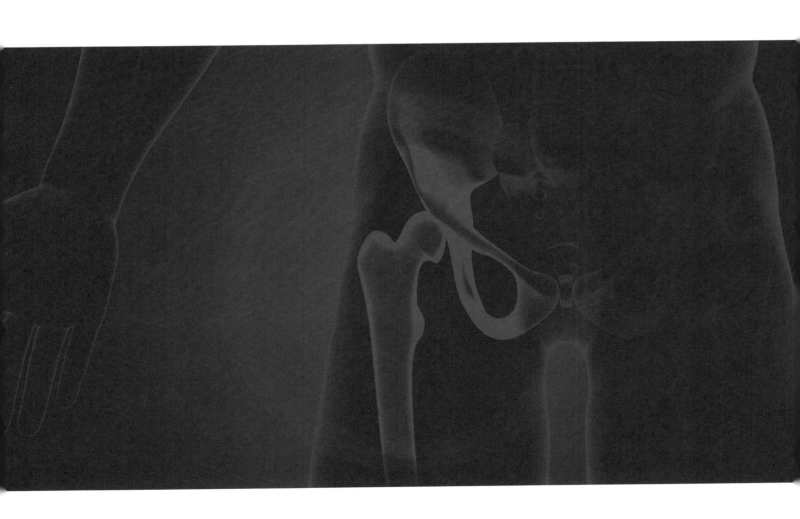

FEMORAL TORSION

- Femoral torsion is the relative rotation (twist) between the femur's shaft and neck. When viewed from above, the femoral neck projects about 15 degrees anterior to the medial-lateral axis through the femoral condyles.
- This 15-degree anterior projection is considered normal and is termed femoral anteversion. Therefore, the patient should present between 8 – 15 degrees of femoral anteversion under normal conditions and without pathology.
- Any additional torsion beyond 15 degrees is termed excessive femoral anteversion. Any torsion less than 8 degrees is termed femoral retroversion or an outward twisting of the femoral neck.

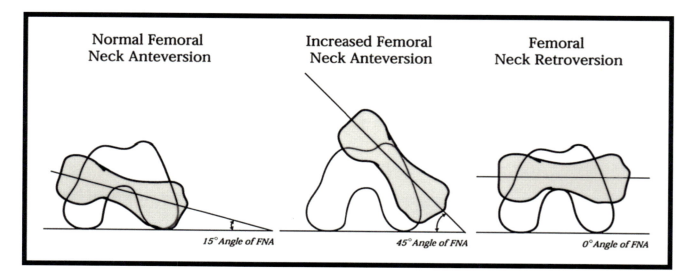

FEMORAL ANTEVERSION

Quick Example:
Parents bring their child to PT because of in-toeing during ambulation.

Findings:
- Classically, the child sits in a W-position.
- Excessive hip internal rotation (>70°)
- Restricted hip external rotation (<20°)
- Genu valgum with increased Q-angle present
- Relative external tibial rotation compensation
- The greater the genu valgum, the greater the subtalar pronation

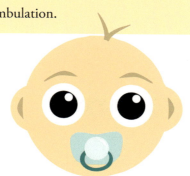

*At birth, normal femoral anteversion is 30-40°, which reduces to 10- 15° by skeletal maturity.

*According to Neuman, any femoral torsion greater than 15 degrees indicates excessive femoral anteversion.

CHAPTER 7

FEMORAL RETROVERSION

Quick Example:
Parents bring their child to PT because of out-toeing during ambulation.

Findings:
- Excessive hip external rotation (>70°)
- Restricted hip internal rotation (<20°)
- Genu varum with medial compartmental pain
- Relative internal tibial rotation compensation

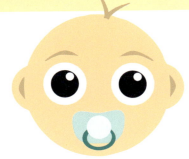

*This structural deformity is relatively uncommon when compared to excessive femoral anteversion.

*According to Neuman, any femoral torsion under 8 degrees indicates excessive femoral retroversion.

"THE PT HUSTLE ISN'T JUST A COMPANY I BUILT; IT'S A WAY OF LIFE. EVERY DAY IS A HUSTLE TO ACHIEVE YOUR WILDEST DREAMS. PT IS WHAT YOU CHOSE AS THE PATH TO GET YOU THERE."

—COACH K

CHAPTER 8

FOOT MECHANICS

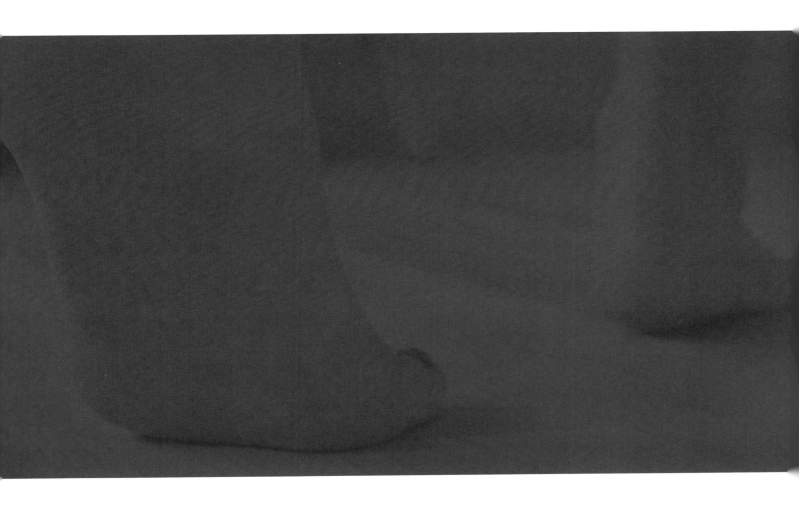

FOREFOOT VARUS

DEFINITION

Forefoot varus is the angling or inverted position of the bones in the front of the foot relative to the heel. Described as the "thumbs up" or "big toe up" position.

> **SPECIAL NPTE NOTES**
> The average amount of forefoot varus is 0 – 10 degrees in normal adults.

A PRINCIPLE TO REMEMBER DURING THE ASSESSMENT

In a closed chain position, the goal of the foot is to remain level with the ground until the toe-off (pre-swing) phase of gait.

Applying the principle above, when the patient presents with excessive forefoot varus, the rearfoot will attempt to evert, forcing the medial forefoot to the ground. This excessive forefoot varus is called "compensated forefoot varus."

TREATMENT FOR EXCESSIVE FOREFOOT VARUS

- When a patient presents with a rigid forefoot varus, the principle is to "bring the ground up to the foot," which means placing a medial wedge into the shoe that fills the gap!
- When a patient presents with a flexible forefoot varus, the principle is to "assist the foot down to the ground," which means adding a lateral wedge that pushes underneath the lateral forefoot, rotating the big toe down to the ground!

CHAPTER 8

FOREFOOT VALGUS[14]

DEFINITION

Forefoot valgus is the angling or everted position of the bones in the front of the foot relative to the heel. Forefoot valgus appears as the "thumbs down" or "big toe down" position.

> **SPECIAL NPTE NOTES**
> This abnormal position is often associated with pes planus (flat foot).

A PRINCIPLE TO REMEMBER DURING TREATMENT

When treating a patient with a foot deformity, always determine if they have a rigid or flexible deformity first.

Flexible and rigid foot deformities are treated differently on the NPTE

Always place the wedge underneath a rigid deformity (i.e., a lateral wedge for a stiff forefoot valgus. Place the wedge on the opposite side (i.e., medial side) for a flexible forefoot valgus.

Don't fret! Apply these same principles to the rearfoot as well! Make sure to check your orthotics textbook and kinesiology textbook for further practice and application of these principles.

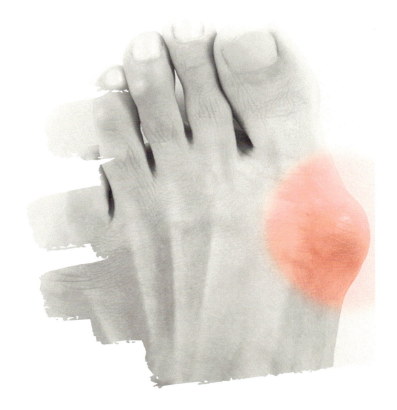

41

"SUCCESS WON'T JUST COME KNOCK ON YOUR DOOR...YOU HAVE TO GO OUT AND GET IT."

–COACH K

CHAPTER 9

GAIT DEVIATIONS

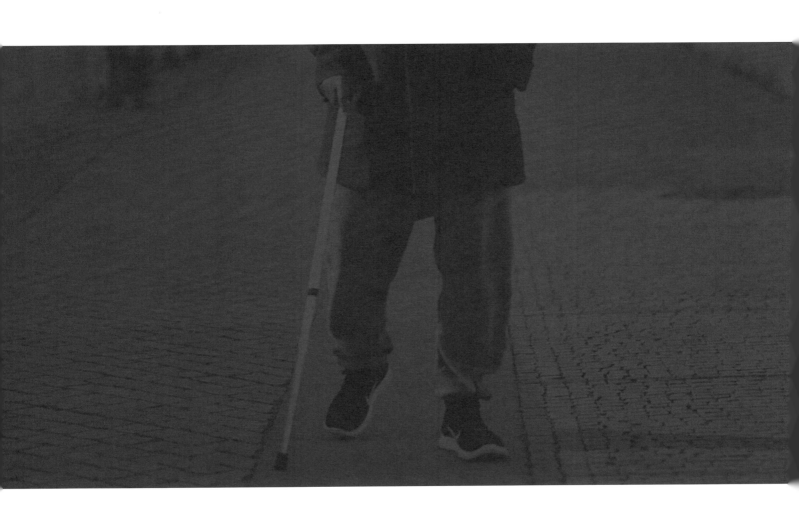

TRICKY GAIT DEVIATIONS[15]

VAULTING

It is a gait deviation characterized by active plantarflexion of the stance limb to clear the contralateral limb during the swing phase.

When does it occur?
During midstance, when using the shorter lower extremity.

Common causes:
- Leg length discrepancy
- Contralateral prosthesis is too long.
- Contralateral foot stuck into plantarflexion.

KNEE THRUST

It is a gait deviation characterized by a rapid hyperextension of the knee. This deviation most often occurs to move the center of mass anterior to the knee, thereby producing a knee extensor moment.

When does it occur?
During loading response to midstance.

Common causes:
- Weak quadriceps
- Spastic quadriceps
- Plantarflexor contracture

TRENDELENBURG

It is a gait deviation characterized by a marked lateral trunk lean towards the weakened lower extremity. This lateral trunk lean shifts the center of mass towards the weak side, decreasing the load on the ipsilateral hip abductors.

When does it occur?
During midstance on the affected side/side of the lateral trunk lean.

Common causes:
- Gluteus medius/minimus weakness
- Ipsilateral hip adductor tightness
- Superior gluteal nerve palsy

CHAPTER 9

DELAYED HEEL OFF

A gait deviation characterized by a lack of plantarflexion resulting in an inability to transfer weight onto the forefoot in preparation for swing.

When does it occur?
During terminal stance to pre-swing

Common causes:
- Weak plantarflexors
- Excessive dorsiflexion mobility
- Tibial nerve palsy
- Anterior foot pain

EARLY HEEL OFF

It is a gait deviation characterized by an inability to achieve adequate dorsiflexion during the late stance phase.

When does it occur?
During Midstance

Common causes:
- Limited posterior talocrural capsular mobility
- Tight or spastic plantarflexors
- Heel pain

BACK WARD TRUNK LEAN

It is a gait deviation characterized by marked trunk extension to shift the center of mass posteriorly and reduce the load on the gluteus maximus.

When does it occur?
During initial contact - midstance

Common causes:
- Gluteus maximus weakness
- Inferior gluteal nerve palsy

"YOU DON'T GET WHAT YOU WANT… YOU GET WHAT YOU ARE."

—MYRON GOLDEN

CHAPTER 10

GOUT

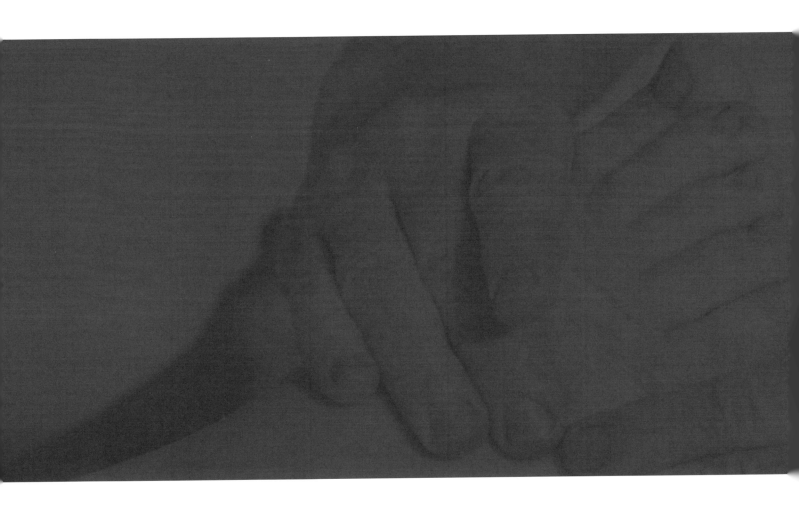

SECTION I

GOUT[16]

- Gout is a monoarticular inflammatory process that develops in some people with high uric acid levels in the blood.
- The uric acid buildup can form needlelike crystals in a joint and cause sudden and severe episodes of pain, redness, warmth, and swelling.

WHO PRIMARILY GETS THIS?

Males over 30 with a purine-rich diet and/or indulge in excessive use of alcohol.

MAJOR CAUSES OF GOUT	
Obesity	A Purine-Rich Diet
Excessive Alcohol Use	Red Meat
Hypothyroidism	Sardines/Anchovies
Renal Disease	Liver
Immune Suppression Drugs	Dried Beans & Peas
Psoriasis	Mushrooms

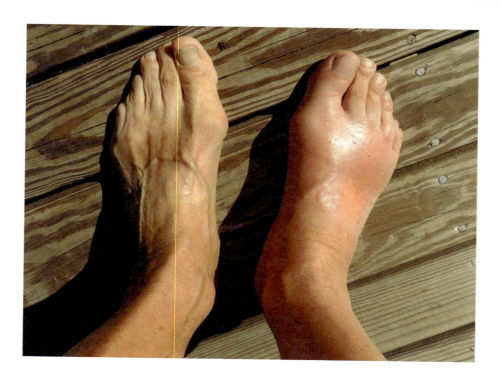

WHAT SHOULD THE PT LOOK OUT FOR?	
LAB VALUES	Hyperuricemia or Elevated Uric Acid in the blood (> 7.0 mg/dL) Males – Uric Acid Normal Range: 3.4-7.0 mg/dL Females – Uric Acid Normal Range: 2.4-6.0 mg/dL
TIME OF ONSET	A patient with an acute onset of gout typically complains of a sudden sharp pain inside the affected joint that **started at night**.
PAIN LOCATIONS	Gout is typically a **monoarticular inflammatory condition that affects the foot's first metatarsophalangeal (MTP)** joint. However, the ankle, instep, knee, wrist/hand, fingers, or elbow can be the site of an initial attack.
SIGNS & SYMPTOMS	"G.O.U.T. T.O.E." **G**REAT TOE PAIN **O**NE JOINT, IN MOST CASES **U**RIC ACID ELEVATED **T**ACHYCARDIA **T**OPHI **O**VERLY SENSITIVE & CHILLS **E**RYTHEMA & FEVER
MEDICATIONS	"C.A.N." **C**OLCHICINE **A**LLOPURINOL **N**SAIDS

"NO MEANINGFUL CHANGE EVER HAPPENS IN A PLACE OF COMFORT AND SECURITY"

–COACH K

CHAPTER 11

HISTORY TAKING

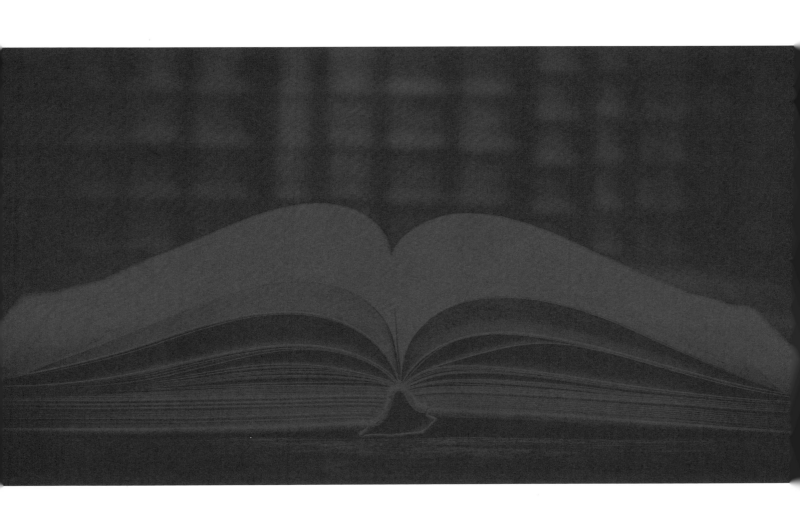

SECTION I

DETERMINING POSSIBLE TISSUES, STRUCTURES, OR SYSTEMS INVOLVED

WAS THERE A TRAUMA THAT OCCURRED (MECHANISM OF INJURY)?

This question allows the therapist to gain some initial direction regarding the potentially injured tissues. Therapists should ask this question early to guide the subjective examination process.

Examples:
Blow to the lateral knee that is flexed and fixed.
- Terrible Triad (i.e., Medial meniscal tear, Medial collateral ligament sprain, & ACL tear)

A sudden and forceful external rotation during shoulder abduction.
- Anterior dislocation

Fall onto an outstretched hand with a pronated forearm (FOOSH).
- Colles fracture

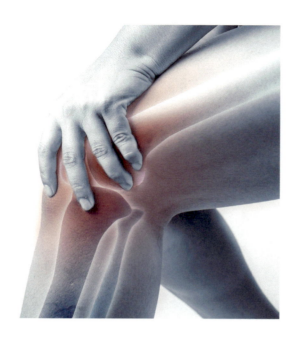

WHAT ARE THE EXACT MOVEMENTS OR ACTIVITIES THAT CAUSE THE PAIN?

This type of question allows the examiner to differentiate whether the pain is musculoskeletal, mechanical, or systemic. This question can also be great to determine whether more questions are required to expose yellow or red flags.

Examples:
Pain reaching overhead between 90 – 120 degrees is consistent with subacromial pathologies.
- Supraspinatus tendinitis/tear or bursitis

Groin pain that is aggravated by crossing the affected leg over the other.
- Flexion, adduction, and internal rotation are consistent with hip labral pathology.

CHAPTER 11

WHAT TYPES OF SENSATIONS DOES THE PATIENT FEEL?

This question allows the therapist to pinpoint the type of injured tissue by understanding the associated pain type.

PAIN DESCRIPTIONS & RELATED STRUCTURES	
Types of Pain	Structure
Cramping, dull, aching	Muscle
Dull, aching	Ligament, joint capsule
Sharp, shooting	Nerve root
Sharp, bright, lightning-like	Nerve
Burning, pressure-like, stinging, aching	Sympathetic nerve
Deep, nagging, dull	Bone
Sharp, severe, intolerable	Fracture
Throbbing, diffuse	Vasculature

DETERMINING THE IRRITABILITY OF THE TISSUE

IS THE PAIN CONSTANT OR INTERMITTENT?

This question is one of the most important and one of the most used. This question allows the therapist to determine the irritability of the tissue and the type of tissue injured.

Constant Pain
- Suggestive of chemical pain, tumors, or visceral pain.

Intermittent Pain
- Suggestive of mechanical or musculoskeletal pain.

The therapist will need to ask more clarifying questions about movements or activities that bring on the pain. Asking more clarification questions can assist with determining the tissue at fault.

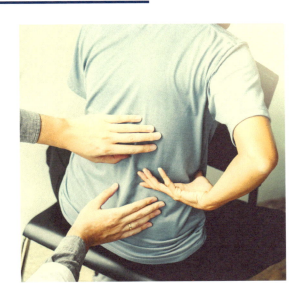

SECTION I

DETERMINING TYPES OF INFLAMMATION

IS THE PAIN ASSOCIATED WITH REST, ACTIVITY, SPECIFIC POSTURES, OR TIME OF DAY?

Determining whether a patient is experiencing inflammation is essential for the NPTE, but you must also determine the acuity.

Examples:

1. Pain on activity that decreases with rest: mechanical pain (e.g., adhesions)

2. Morning pain that improves with activity: chronic inflammation (e.g., osteoarthritis)

3. Pain or aching as day progresses: joint swelling/congestion

4. Pain at rest and worse at the beginning of activity as compared to the end: Acute inflammation

5. Pain that is not affected by rest or activity: bone or systemic pain

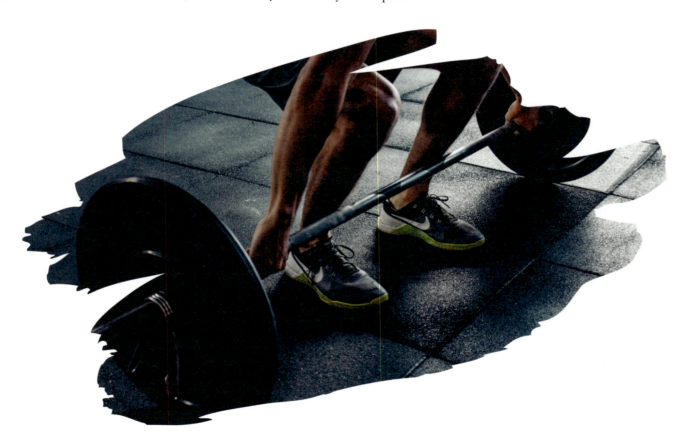

"LOOK FOR SOMETHING POSITIVE EACH DAY, EVEN IF SOME DAYS YOU HAVE TO LOOK A BIT HARDER."

—COACH K

CHAPTER 12

INNOMINATE ROTATIONS

SECTION I

INNOMINATE ROTATIONS & MUSCLE ENERGY TECHNIQUES

BACKGROUND

Pelvic innominate rotations are a type of musculoskeletal dysfunction that occurs at the SIJ and can cause pelvic malalignment, pain, and long-term mechanical problems. These innominate rotations are tested on the NPTE using the Supine-to-Sit test.

The Supine-to-Sit test is a special test used to identify the presence of an anteriorly or posteriorly rotated innominate. Determining the type of rotation present is vital to determining proper treatment.

HOW THE TEST WORKS

With the patient lying supine, the length of each leg is compared by looking at the resting positions of the medial malleoli bilaterally.

The patient is then asked to transition into long sitting from supine, and the length of each leg is compared by looking at the resting positions of the medial malleoli bilaterally.

Condition 1: If the right leg appears longer than the left in supine and then appears shorter than the left in long sitting, the patient is said to have a right anterior innominate rotation.

Condition 2: If the right leg appears shorter than the left in supine and then appears longer than the left in long sitting, the patient is said to have a right posterior innominate rotation.

MNEUMONIC

"All patients with ALS (Amyotrophic Lateral Sclerosis) need SLP (Speech-Language Pathology)."

You are observing an **A**NTERIOR INNOMINATE ROTATION

if the tested leg goes from **L**ONG

to **S**HORT

CHAPTER 12

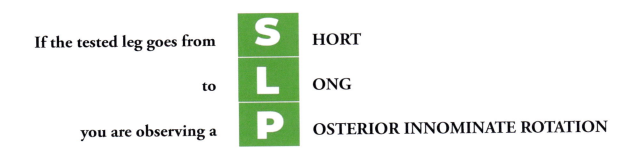

If the tested leg goes from **SHORT** to **LONG** you are observing a **POSTERIOR INNOMINATE ROTATION**

TREATING INNOMINATE ROTATIONS, THE NPTE WAY

Treating innominate rotations on the NPTE can be very tricky but straightforward. The basis of your decision-making relies on which way the innominate is rotated. YOU MUST DETERMINE THIS FIRST!

After determining the rotation, consider the muscles that can return the innominate to its original position. For example, if you have a right posteriorly innominate rotation, you must have the patient contract a muscle that will anteriorly rotate the right innominate.

Which muscle can do that?
THE HIP FLEXORS!

Let's give you another example. Which intervention would be best if you have a patient with a known left anteriorly rotated innominate?

Since we know the left side is anteriorly rotated, we must select a muscle group that can posteriorly rotate the left innominate.

Which muscle can do that?
THE HAMSTRINGS!

Although the hamstrings are not the only muscle group that can posteriorly rotate the innominate, we can perform an exercise such as single leg bridging to treat this pelvic dysfunction appropriately.

CHAPTER 13

ISOKINETIC TESTING

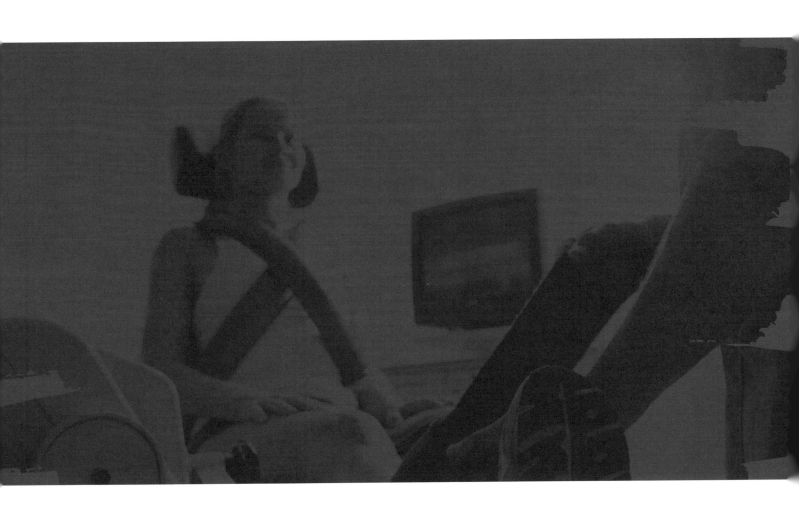

SECTION I

ISOKINETIC DYNAMOMETRY[17]

THE BASICS

Isokinetic testing, which in Latin means **reacting at the same rate**, is a common form of dynamic strength testing performed with an isokinetic dynamometer.

Isokinetic testing **is performed on most major muscle groups** and **maintains a constant angular velocity while measuring the external torque applied to resist the patient's produced internal torque.**

HOW IT WORKS

The clinician determines the speed at which the patient will work during the strength assessment. The isokinetic dynamometer device will dynamically adjust its resistance to match the patient's force production. This force-match feature keeps the patient moving at that same speed through the range of motion.

WHEN TO USE

The isokinetic dynamometer can assess strength at different ranges of motion and certain speeds. This tool can help determine the strength of a muscle, muscle function, and likelihood of muscle injury. **This device is often used with the athletic population for return-to-sport strength assessments.**

BONUS: ISOKINETIC EXERCISES

It can be challenging to distinguish isokinetic and isotonic exercises on practice exams when preparing for the NPTE.

Remember, isokinetic is the same speed and variable resistance, while isotonic is the same resistance and variable speeds.

- **Treadmill at a predetermined speed**
- **Step/Stairmaster at a predetermined selected speed**
- **Stationary bike**
- **Upper or lower body ergometer**
- **Biodex machine (Isokinetic device)**

"SOMETIMES YOU WIN AND SOMETIMES YOU LEARN."

–COACH K

CHAPTER 14

LUMBAR MECHANICAL TRACTION

SECTION I

LUMBAR MECHANICAL TRACTION DURATION AND FORCE[18]

LUMBAR MECHANICAL TRACTION (MT)

The process of applying a stretching force to the lumbar vertebrae through body weight, weights, and/or pulleys to distract individual joints of the lumbar spine.

5 KEY PRINCIPLES FOR DECISION-MAKING

1. Friction created by the patient's body on the traction table MUST BE overcome to produce movement at the lumbar spine. **Greater than 25% is required to overcome friction.**

2. High poundage, **greater than 50% of the patient's body weight, is required to achieve separation of joint spaces in the lumbar spine.**

3. When attempting lumbar MT for the first time, **a maximum of 30lbs should be trialed to determine patient response.**

4. **In the acute phase, patients may tolerate traction**; however, the duration should be **less than 15 minutes for intermittent lumbar MT** and **less than 10 minutes for sustained lumbar mechanical traction.**

5. **Maximum duration of lumbar MT should be 30 minutes.** A longer duration is appropriate with the subacute/chronic phases and when the patient reports progressive symptom improvement.

CHAPTER 14

5 KEY STEPS FOR DECISION-MAKING

Step 1: Is my patient appropriate for lumbar mechanical traction?
Patients with unremitting pain, lumbar spine instability, and/or cancer are not candidates for lumbar MT.

Step 2: Does my patient have an exaggeration of symptoms with lumbar movement?
Physical therapists should trial sustained lumbar MT for patients who have pain with lumbar movement instead of intermittent lumbar (MT)

Step 3: Is this my patient's first time using lumbar (MT)?
Physical therapists should trial a maximum of 30 lbs. of force for first-time users of lumbar mechanical traction.

Step 4: Which phase of healing is my patient in?
Patients in the acute phase should slowly progress in force, beginning at a maximum of 30 lbs. and progressing to 25%, 30%, and so forth. The duration should last no longer than 15 minutes for intermittent lumbar MT.

Step 5: Does my patient have a compressive spinal condition and respond well to traction? (e.g., spinal stenosis, facet compression)

*Patients in the subacute phase with compressive lumbar conditions that respond well to traction should progress to greater than 50% force for up to 30 minutes.

CHAPTER 15

MEDIAL MENISCAL TEAR

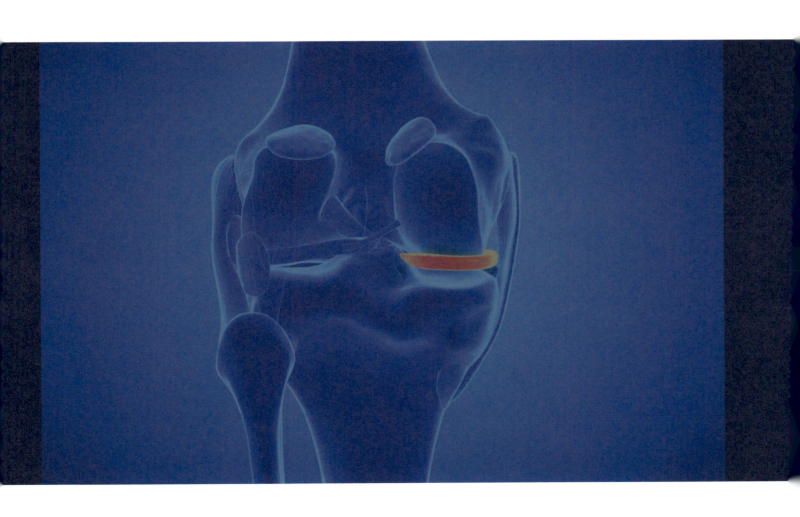

SECTION I

TOP 5 FACTS FOR MEDIAL MENISCAL TEARS[19]

ANATOMY

The medial meniscus is firmly attached to the joint capsule, MCL, ACL, PCL, and semimembranosus.

Dr. Rice's NPTE Pearl: Since the medial meniscus has several attachments to other commonly injured soft tissues, the medial meniscus is often the correct answer if it is between lateral and medial meniscal tears.

HEALING

Since the peripheral 1/3rd of the meniscus is vascularized, tears that occur in this region have a high healing potential. Tears in the deeper and inner 2/3rds are considered avascular and don't heal well. These tears often require surgery.

Dr. Rice's NPTE Pearl: If there is a diagnosed medial meniscal tear at the peripheral 1/3rd, conservative treatment is most likely before resorting to surgery. Focus on reducing the acuteness of the condition with modalities and light mobility-based exercises. AVOID deep squats or pivoting on the affected knee.

MECHANISM OF INJURY

Medial meniscal tears are commonly injured during a pivot on a planted foot, widely seen in sports, or stepping into a hole in the ground. Several attachments to the medial meniscus make it vulnerable to injuries from hyperextension and traumatic blows to the medial or lateral knee.

CLINICAL PRESENTATION

Mild to severe pain with intermittent clicking and popping is present with ambulation or general knee movement. Occasional "catching" at specific parts of the range is also a common finding.

Dr. Rice's NPTE Pearl: Most other traumatic knee injuries do not present with clicking or popping inside the joint. On the NPTE, because crepitus can be confused with popping/clicking, it would be wise to clear osteoarthritis as an option.

SPECIAL TESTS

Apley's and **McMurray's** tests are two standard NPTE special tests used to identify meniscal tears. These two tests attempt to compress the knee while rotating (i.e., creating shear) to elicit pain, clicking, and/or popping.

INCREDIBLE OFFER OPPORTUNITY

Are you ready to ace the NPTE and kickstart your career as a Physical Therapist? Join over 20,000 Physical Therapy graduates who have trusted Coach K's NPTE review courses and coaching programs to guide them to success.

Under Coach K's expert guidance, you'll discover the proven formula for answering every type of NPTE question with confidence. No need to spend endless hours studying—Coach K's program is designed to make your prep efficient and effective.

Don't miss out! Limited spots are available, so act fast and scan the QR code below for more information and secure your spot in this all-inclusive program.

Your dream PT career is just one step away!

CHAPTER 16

MSK BREATHING MECHANICS

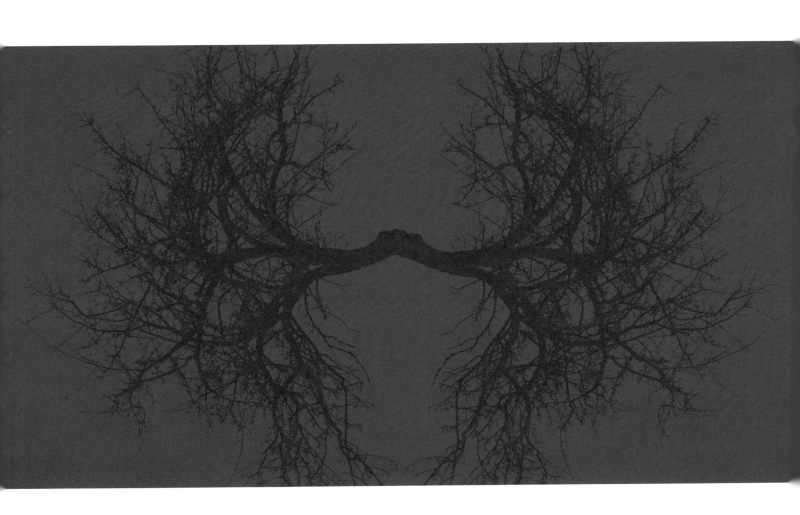

BASIC MECHANICS OF THE UPPER RIBS

- Ribs 1 - 6 are a part of the upper ribs.
- This set of ribs has more anterior and forward movement during inspiration compared to ribs 7 -12.
- The movement of the first six ribs during inspiration & expiration is comparable to that of a pump handle (*like the one used to pump gasoline*).

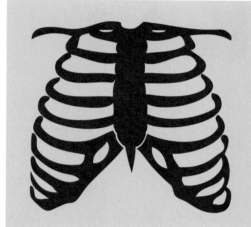

The primary joint motion that occurs during inspiration & expiration is at the costovertebral (CV) joints.

During Inspiration: An anterior and superior roll of ribs 1 - 6 with an associated inferior glide at each CV joint.

During Expiration: A posterior and inferior roll of ribs 1 - 6 with an associated superior glide at each CV joint.

MOBILIZING TO IMPROVE BREATHING MECHANICS OF UPPER RIBS (CV JOINTS)[20]

TO IMPROVE **INHALATION**:

Inferior glides **I**mprove **I**nhalation

TO IMPROVE **EXHALATION**:

Superior glides **I**mprove **E**xhalation

MUSCLES & INNERVATIONS OF QUIET INSPIRATION

Diaphragm
- Increases the vertical diameter of the thorax by transitioning from a dome shape to a flattened shape during contraction.
- Innervated by the Phrenic Nerve (C3-C5)

Scalenes
- Increases intrathoracic volume by elevating the ribs and sternum.
- Innervated by the Ventral rami of spinal roots (C3-C7)

Intercostales Externi
- Increases intrathoracic volume by elevating the ribs and expanding the chest cavity.
- Innervated by the Intercostal Nerves (T2-T12)

MUSCLES AND INNERVATIONS OF FORCED EXPIRATION

Abdominals
- Decrease intrathoracic volume by flexing the trunk and depressing the ribs.
- Push the diaphragm upwards.
- Innervated by the Intercostal Nerves (T7-L1)

Intercostales Interni
- Decreases intrathoracic volume by depressing the ribs.
- Innervated by the Intercostal Nerves (T2-T12)

"EVERYTHING SEEMS IMPOSSIBLE UNTIL IT'S DONE..."

#FACTS

CHAPTER 17

MUSCULOSKELETAL DIAGNOSTIC IMAGING

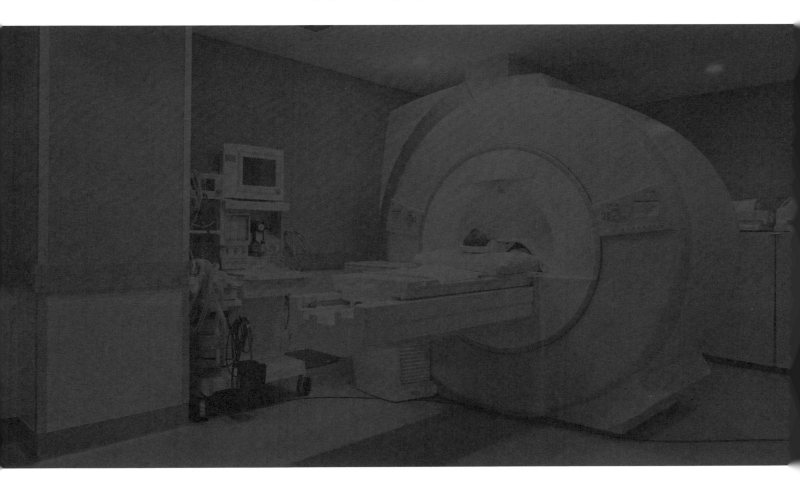

SECTION I

DIAGNOSTIC IMAGING TYPES

X-RAY RADIOGRAPHIC IMAGING

Using ionizing electromagnetic radiation to pass through body tissues produces an image of attenuated structures.

Clinical Notes:
- Radiographs are often considered the best initial study for musculoskeletal disorders.
- Medical professionals often use radiographs for initial joint, spine, and cardiopulmonary disease assessments.

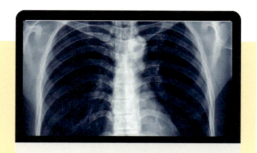

COMPUTERIZED TOMOGRAPHY (CT-SCAN)[21]

The medical community employs ionizing electromagnetic radiation from different angles, using multiple X-rays, to produce cross-sectional body slices.

Clinical Uses of CT-Scan Examples
1. Subtle or complex fractures
2. Central spinal stenosis
3. First imaging choice in severe trauma involving multiple bone and soft tissue injuries.

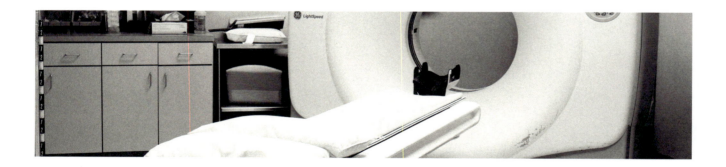

CHAPTER 17

BONE SCINTIGRAPHY (BONE SCAN)

A nuclear imaging test that uses ionizing radiation and a small amount of radioactive nucleotide to assess for bone disease.

Clinical Uses of A Bone Scan Examples
- Localizing bone tumors
- Detecting skeletal metastasis
- Early diagnosis of stress fractures

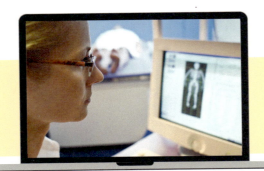

MAGNETIC RESONANCE IMAGING (MRI)[22]

Medical professionals utilize nuclear magnetic resonance to visualize tissues within the body. The MRI technique does not use ionizing radiation, distinguishing it from radiographs and CT and PET scans.

Clinical Uses of MRI Examples
1. Rotator cuff tears & muscular disorders (e.g., atrophy, strains)
2. Meniscal & labral abnormalities
3. Neurologic conditions (entrapment, compression)
4. Disc herniations and causes of nerve root compression
5. Variations in bone marrow (e.g., stress fracture, bone tumors, avascular necrosis)

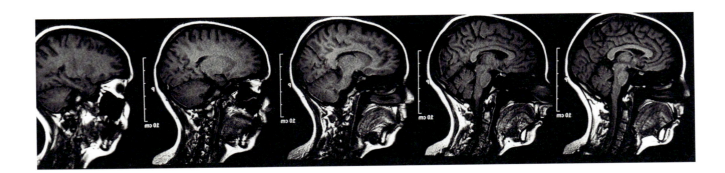

"THIS IS JUST ANOTHER CHAPTER IN YOUR LIFE, NOT THE END OF YOUR STORY."

—COACH K

CHAPTER 18

PLUMB LINE

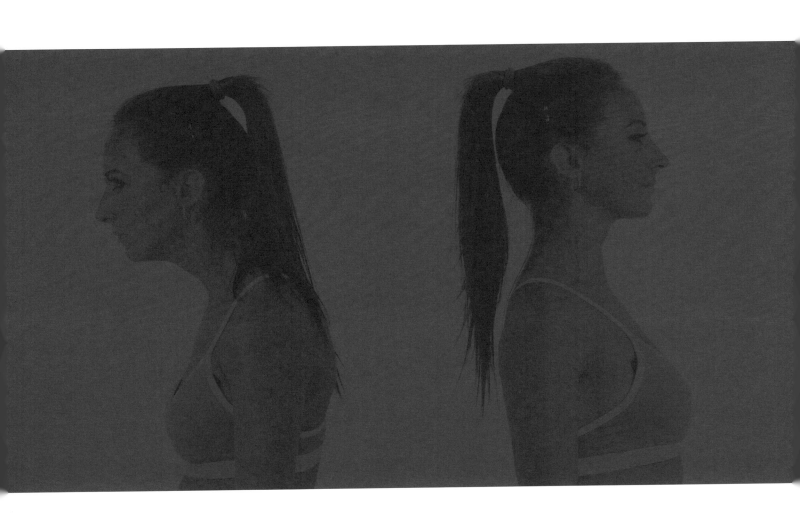

POSTURAL ASSESSMENT[23]

NPTE JOINTS TO KNOW	LINE OF GRAVITY (WHERE THE PLUMB LINE SHOULD FALL)	ACTIVE MUSCLES
Alanto-Occipital Joint	Anterior	Suboccipitals & Cervical Extensors
Cervical Joint	Posterior	Anterior Scalene and deep Neck Flexors
Thoracic Joint	Anterior	Erector Spinae (Thoracis)
Lumbar Joint	Posterior	Abdominals
Sacroiliac Joint	Anterior	Transverse Abdominus (TA)
Hip Joint	Posterior	Iliopsoas
Knee Joint	Anterior	Hamstrings & Gastrocnemius
Ankle Joint	Anterior	Plantarflexors

"WORK HARD, DREAM BIG."

–COACH K

CHAPTER 19

PROSTHETIC GAIT DEVIATIONS

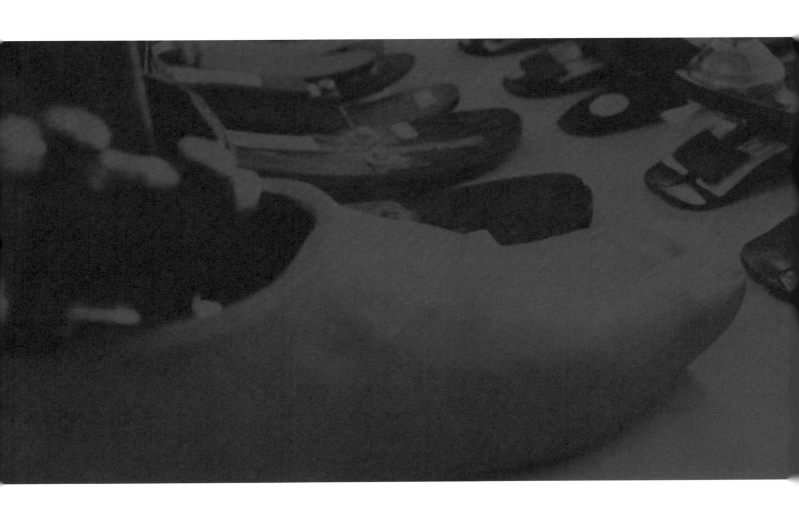

SECTION 1

TOP 3 TRANSTIBIAL PROSTHETIC GAIT DEVIATIONS

1) EXCESSIVE KNEE EXTENSION DURING INITIAL CONTACT TO LOADING RESPONSE[25]

What should happen in this phase?

In the normal gait pattern, using a transtibial prosthesis, the knee should flex smoothly between 8 to 10 degrees during initial contact to loading response. This knee flexion allows for weight acceptance and proper absorption of ground forces.

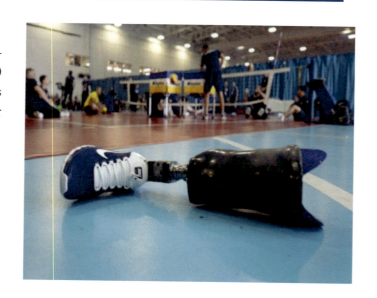

What is the gait deviation?

During initial contact to loading response, while observing from the side, the patient keeps the knee extended on the prosthetic side. This extension makes the limb longer, reduces shock absorption, and increases energy expenditure.

What does the patient complain about?

1. Sensation of walking uphill

2. Anterior distal stump pain

What are the Top 2 NPTE causes to know?

Too Soft Cushioned Heel
A too-soft heel wedge (cushioned heel) allows the prosthetic foot to plantarflex too quickly. This premature contact of the entire foot with the ground extends the knee. *Think about your biomechanics: Ankle plantarflexion promotes knee extension, and ankle dorsiflexion promotes knee flexion.

Posteriorly Displaced Socket or Anteriorly Set Prosthetic Foot
A posteriorly displaced socket sets the knee posterior to the foot during the initial contact to loading response. During the loading response, as the patient shifts weight onto the foot, the line of gravity moves to a position anterior to the knee. This is known as an extensor moment and creates extension at the knee.

CHAPTER 19

2) KNEE INSTABILITY DURING INITIAL CONTACT TO LOADING RESPONSE[26]

What should happen in this phase?

In the normal gait pattern, using a transtibial prosthesis, the knee should flex smoothly between 8 to 10 degrees during initial contact to loading response. This knee flexion allows for weight acceptance and proper absorption of ground forces.

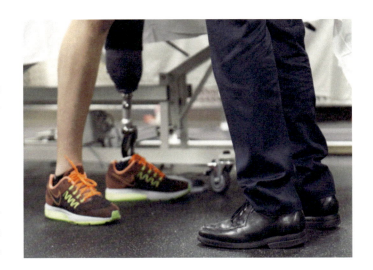

What is the gait deviation?

During initial contact to loading response, while observing from the side, the patient buckles into knee flexion or avoids buckling by shortening the stance time. A smooth, energy-efficient gait requires good stability at the knee.

What does the patient complain about?

1. Knee buckling or feeling unstable

2. Fear of falling

What are the Top 2 NPTE causes to know?

Too hard Cushioned Heel
A too-hard heel wedge (cushioned heel) does not allow for adequate plantarflexion of the prosthetic foot during loading response. Because of the lack of plantarflexion, the patient loses shock absorption and compensates by flexing at the knee to get the foot down onto the floor. *Think about your biomechanics: Ankle plantarflexion promotes knee extension, and ankle dorsiflexion promotes knee flexion.

Anteriorly Displaced Socket or Posteriorly Set Prosthetic Foot
An anteriorly displaced socket sets the knee more anterior than the foot during initial contact to loading response. As the patient shifts their weight onto the prosthetic foot, the line of gravity moves to a position posterior to the knee. This flexor moment can create excessive flexion (buckling) at the knee.

3) WIDE BASED GAIT DURING MIDSTANCE

What should happen in this phase?

In normal midstance, the transtibial prosthesis is positioned in relative extension when supporting the entire body weight on a single limb. The pelvis should be level, and the patient's trunk should be relatively neutral in the frontal plane.

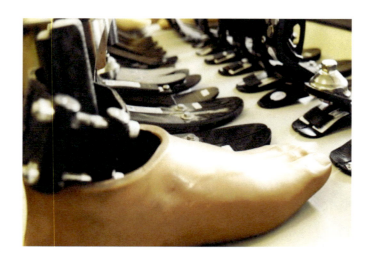

What is the gait deviation?

During midstance, as one places the prosthetic limb more laterally, the base of support also moves more laterally. One accomplishes this gait deviation by abducting the hip on the prosthetic side. This deviation from normal causes increased energy expenditure and medial instability.

What does the patient complain about?

1. Pain at the proximal lateral brim of the socket

2. Pain at the medial distal end of the residual limb

What are the Top 2 NPTE causes to know?

Outset Foot
Usually, the foot is set 1 cm medial to the center line of the posterior aspect of the socket. Setting the foot too laterally causes the patient to lose medial support. This deviation causes the patient to display a wide-based gait to compensate.

Medially leaning Pylon
The pylon is the prosthesis part that connects the foot to the socket. A medially leaning pylon is when the top of the pylon is displaced more medial than the bottom. When this malalignment occurs, the patient loses medial support, just as in the "Outset foot" case. The patient then produces a wide-based gait during midstance to compensate for the medial instability.

CHAPTER 20

REVERSE MUSCLE ACTIONS

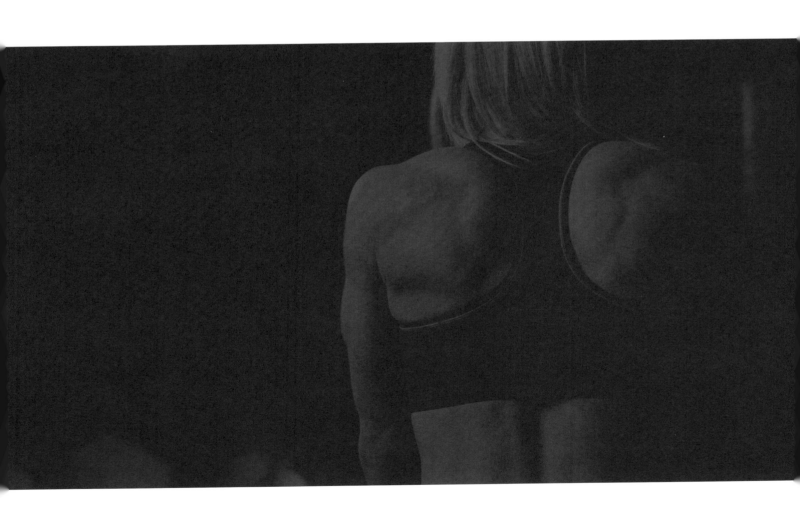

SECTION I

FOUNDATIONAL KNOWLEDGE

OPEN KINETIC CHAIN (OKC) EXERCISE

In physical therapy, we classify an open-chain exercise as a movement in which the distal segment is free to move or when one attaches the distal segment to a movable object.

OKC EXERCISE EXAMPLES
- Lat pull down
- Bench press
- Bicep curls
- Leg press (i.e., plate slides)

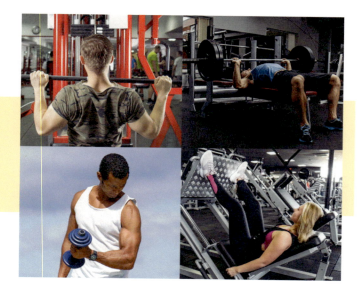

CLOSED KINETIC CHAIN (CKC) EXERCISE

In physical therapy, we define a closed-chain exercise as a movement where either the distal segment remains fixed, or one attaches it to a stationary object.

CKC EXERCISE EXAMPLES
- Squats
- Push-ups
- Pull-ups
- Lunges

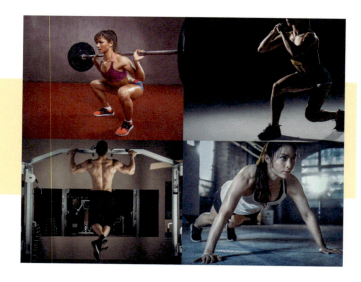

CHAPTER 20

REVERSE MUSCLE ACTIONS[27]

What is a reverse muscle action?

When describing muscle actions, the muscle's insertion point moves toward its origin point.

For example, during elbow flexion, contraction of the long head of the biceps moves the radial tuberosity (i.e., insertion) closer to the fixed supraglenoid tubercle (i.e., origin).

A reverse muscle action occurs when a muscle takes on a different role/action because the **muscle's origin now moves towards a fixed insertion**.

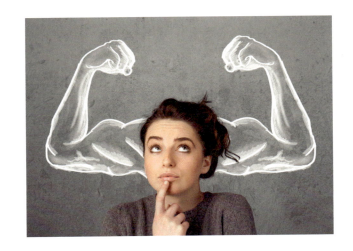

EXAMPLES TO KNOW FOR THE NPTE

BICEPS

- In open chain bicep curls, the long head of the biceps participates in elbow flexion **with the shoulder in neutral (i.e., arm at side)**.
- In closed chain pull-ups, the long head of the biceps contracts, bringing the origin (i.e., supraglenoid tubercle) towards the fixed insertion (i.e., radial tuberosity). This contraction results in elbow flexion **with shoulder extension**.

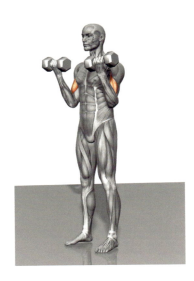

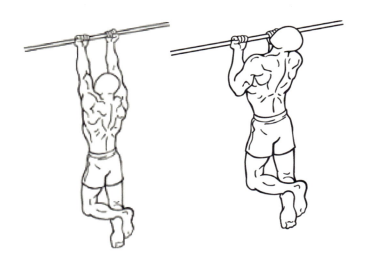

101

MIDDLE DELTOID

- In open-chain shoulder abduction, the participatory muscle is the **middle deltoid**.
- In closed chain shoulder abduction, such as when you perform shoulder abduction isometrically against a wall, the middle deltoid contracts, bringing the origin (i.e., scapular spine) towards the fixed insertion (i.e., deltoid tuberosity). **This contraction causes scapular downward rotation**.

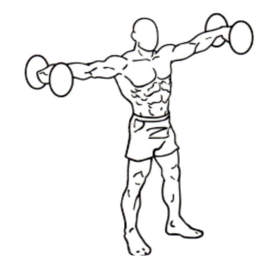

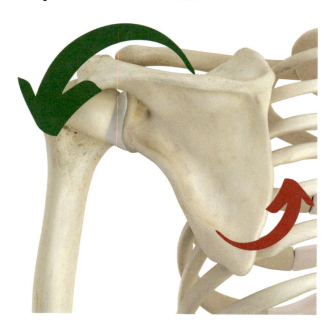

LATISSIMUS DORSI

- The latissimus dorsi participates in shoulder extension, adduction, and internal rotation in open-chain lat pull-downs.
- While engaging in closed-chain 'push-up' pressure relief activities, one can observe that the latissimus dorsi contracts. This action brings the origin, the iliac crest/sacrum, towards the fixed insertion or the floor of the intertubercular groove, resulting in scapular depression and pelvic elevation. These actions lift the buttocks.

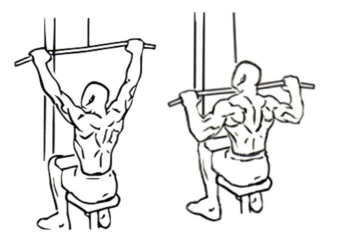

"IF YOU CAN READ THIS...
YOUR BEST DAYS ARE STILL
AHEAD OF YOU."

–COACH K

CHAPTER 21

RHEUMATOID & OSTEO ARTHRITIS

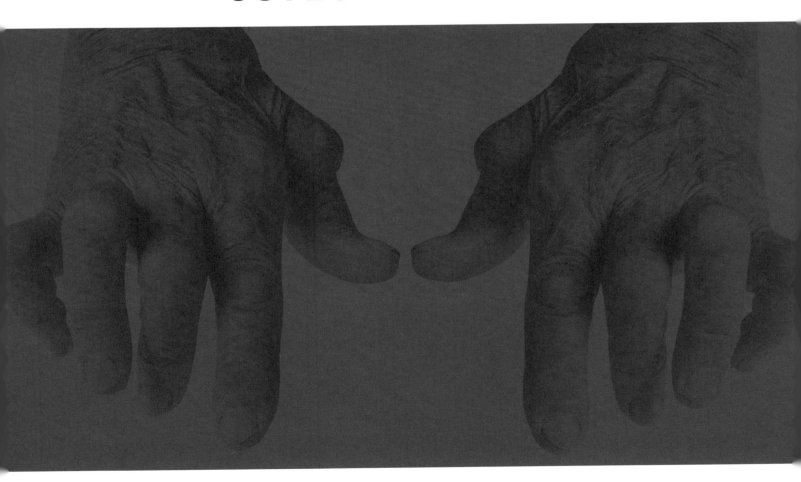

RHEUMATOID ARTHRITIS (RA) VS OSTEOARTHRITIS (OA)[28]

NPTE DIFFERENTIAL CHARACTERISTICS	RA	OA
Pathophysiology	Autoimmune condition, chronic, inflammatory, systemic disease that attacks the synovial lining of joints	Degenerative wear and tear of a joint or joints due to prolonged or repetitive mechanical stress.
Physiological Changes	Inflammatory synovitis with permanent joint structural changes	Cartilage degeneration, Osteophyte formation
Typical Age of Onset	15 – 50+	40+
Onset & Progression	Exacerbations (flare-ups) and remissions are common and can develop suddenly and last weeks to months.	Typically, it develops insidiously (gradually) over the years and worsens over time.
Symmetry	Symmetrical (symptoms occur on both sides of the body)	Asymmetrical
Signs & Symptoms	Redness, warmth, swollen & enlarged joints, prolonged morning stiffness (>45 min.), increased joint pain with activity/weight-bearing. *RA also presents systemic-related symptoms, including fatigue, malaise, fever, weight loss, and multi-system dysfunction	Morning stiffness (<30 min.), increased joint pain with weight-bearing, shear forces, strenuous activity, crepitus or clicking, decreased ROM.
NPTE "Extra Need to Know" Differences	Patients may exhibit ulnar drift of the hands and digits and Swan-neck and Boutonniere deformities, accompanied by rheumatic nodules. Wrist and MCP/MTP joints are often affected.	The possible presence of Heberden's Nodes (DIP) and Bouchard's Nodes (PIP)

"WILL YOUR FUTURE SELF ONE YEAR FROM NOW THANK YOU FOR WHAT YOU'RE DOING TODAY?"

–COACH K

CHAPTER 22

SHIN PAIN

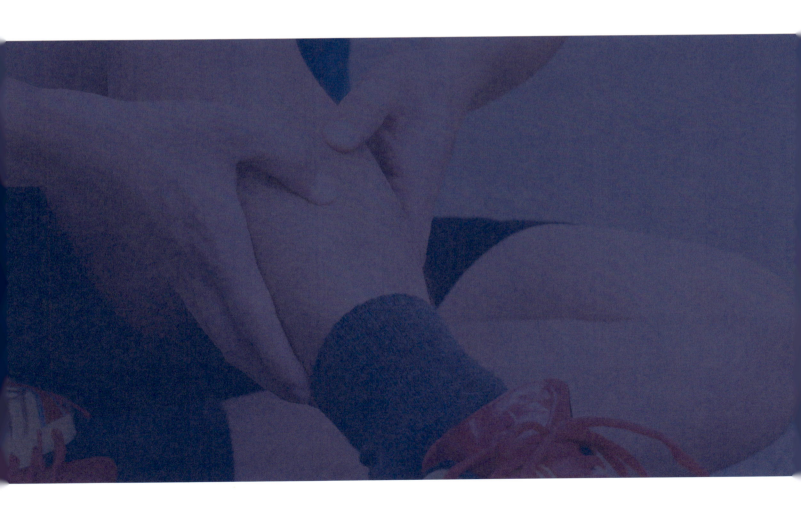

SHIN SPLINTS[29]

Medical professionals also refer to shin splints as medial tibial stress syndrome, manifesting as exercise-induced pain along the distal third of the posteromedial tibial border.

SHIN SPLINTS CLINICAL PROFILE

Mechanism of Injury

- Overuse, repetitive loading stress (i.e., jumping, running).

Pain Type

- Dull pain that is non-focal and extends >5cm in length.

Pain Characteristics

- Pain with stretching and pain present at the beginning of the workout improves with exercise and returns during cool-down.

Range of Motion

- Limited mobility is secondary to tightness in the posterior compartment (i.e., gastrocnemius, soleus, posterior tibialis).

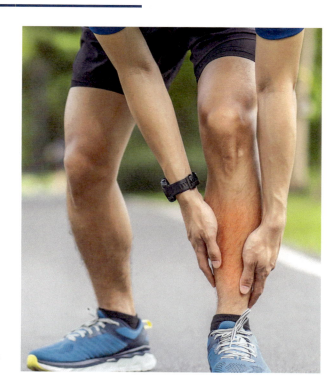

CHAPTER 22

STRESS FRACTURE

On the NPTE, one can also refer to a stress fracture as a ***stress reaction***, a small bone crack resulting from repetitive trauma or loading.

STRESS FRACTURE CLINICAL PROFILE

Mechanism of Injury

- Overuse, repetitive loading stress (i.e., jumping, running)

Pain Type

- Patients often describe a focal deep pain accompanied by point tenderness less than 5 cm in length.

Pain Characteristics

- Pain that is present at rest (especially at night) and with activity.

Range of Motion

- No changes to the range of motion.

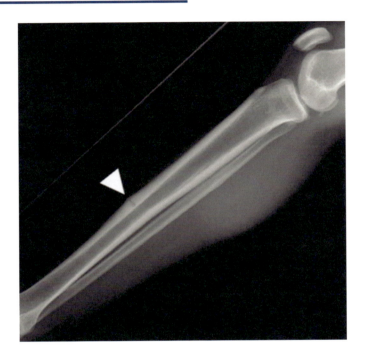

> ***SPECIAL NOTE***
> On the NPTE, when trying to distinguish between a stress fracture and shin splints, look for the results of the palpation exam. Stress fractures are focal pain < 5cm long, and shin splints are non-focal and > 5cm long.

ACUTE COMPARTMENT SYNDROME

This condition is a medical emergency where pressure in the anterior compartment of the lower leg builds up to a dangerous level. This pressure can reduce blood flow, causing death to both neural and musculoskeletal tissues.

ACUTE COMPARTMENT SYNDROME CLINICAL PROFILE

Mechanism of Injury

- Incidents like a broken leg or car accident can cause severe trauma to the anterior compartment.

Pain Type

- Patients often report severe pain, accompanied by sensations of tightness, fullness, numbness, burning, and/or tingling, also known as paresthesia.

Pain Characteristics

- Pain significantly worsens with stretching and is present during rest and activity.

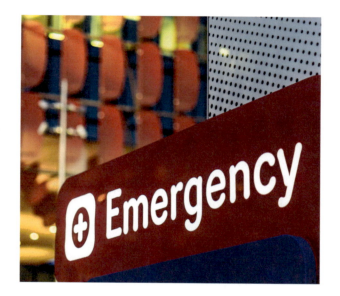

Range of Motion

- Significant changes in ankle mobility are secondary to pain and muscular tightness.

SPECIAL NOTE
Remember, when examining acute compartment syndrome, you may be unable to palpate a dorsal pedal pulse, and also, unlike other musculoskeletal causes of shin pain, acute compartment syndrome can produce neurologic signs/symptoms.

"HAVE YOU EVER ADMIRED THE STARS IN SPACE? IT'S INTERESTING HOW WHEN YOU LOOK CLOSELY, YOU CAN ALWAYS FIND SOMETHING BEAUTIFUL IN A PERIOD OF DARKNESS."

–COACH K

CHAPTER 23

SHOULDER SPECIAL TESTS

SECTION I

PATHOLOGY	SPECIAL TEST(S)	TECHNIQUE	POSITIVE RESULT
Rotator Cuff Full-Thickness Supraspinatus Tear (Grade 3)	Drop-Arm Test	In standing, the patient's arm is passively abducted to 90 degrees. The patient is asked to lower the arm down to the side slowly.	Sudden dropping of the arm due to weakness and an inability to control descent without a report of pain.
Rotator Cuff Full-Thickness Supraspinatus Tear (Grade 1 or 2)	Empty Can Or Jobe Test	(1) In standing, the patient's arm is passively abducted to 90 degrees with no rotation. Resistance is applied in this position. (2) The patient's arm is medially rotated and placed into the scapular plane (empty can), where the thumb is perpendicular to the floor. Downward-directed resistance is then applied.	Pain or weakness is observed when the patient is resisted in the empty can position.
Subacromial Impingement	Hawkens-Kennedy Test	In standing or sitting, the patient's arm is passively brought into 90 degrees of shoulder flexion with the elbow flexed to 90 degrees. The patient's arm is then brought passively into internal rotation.	The patient experiences pain with internal rotation of the shoulder.
	Neer's Test	In standing, the patient's scapula is stabilized with one hand, while the shoulder is internally rotated and passively flexed to the end range.	The patient experiences pain with passive shoulder flexion and internal rotation.

SLAP Tear (Labrum)	Active Compression Test Of O'Brien	In standing or sitting, the patient's arm is placed into 90-degree shoulder flexion and 10-15 degrees horizontal adduction. The patient then fully internally rotates the shoulder and pronates the elbow. (1) A downward force is applied to the arm in this position. (2) The downward force is then applied with the neutral shoulder and forearm position.	Pain reproduction, clicking in the shoulder with the first position and reduced/absent with the second position.
Posterior-Inferior Labral Tear	Kim Test	In supported sitting, the arm is abducted to 90 degrees with the elbow supported in 90 degrees flexion. While supporting the elbow and forearm, the examiner's hand applies an axial compression force to the glenoid through the humerus. While maintaining the axial compression force, the arm is elevated diagonally upward using the same hand, while the other hand applies downward and backward pressure to the proximal arm.	A sudden onset of posterior shoulder pain and clicking is present.
Anterior Dislocation (Anterior Capsular Laxity)	Apprehension Test	In supine, the patient's shoulder is abducted to 90 degrees with 90 degrees of elbow flexion and laterally rotated slowly to end range.	The patient looks or feels apprehensive or alarmed and resists further motion.

AC Joint Degeneration	Cross-Body Adduction Test	(1) The patient's shoulder is flexed to 90 degrees in sitting or standing, followed by a maximal adduction. (2) Bring the tested arm/hand toward the opposite shoulder.	Pain during the adduction or localized pain in the AC joint.
Biceps Tendinitis	Speed's Test	In standing, the patient's shoulder is flexed to 90 degrees, externally rotated, and elbow extended. The examiner applies a downward resistance.	Pain in the bicipital tendon or bicipital groove is reproduced.

"MOST OF US GETTING INTO PHYSICAL THERAPY WANT TO HELP PEOPLE...BUT FIRST, WE NEED TO LEARN HOW TO HELP OURSELVES."

–COACH K

CHAPTER 24

SLAP TEAR ORTHOPEDIC PROTOCOL

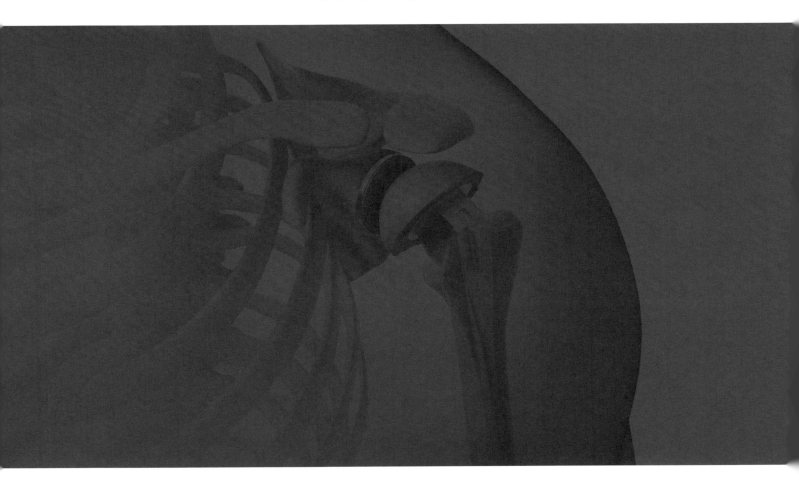

SECTION I

SLAP TEAR REPAIR[31]

In physical therapy, we classify a superior labrum tear as a SLAP lesion that extends anterior to posterior. A type 2 SLAP tear is the most common type, characterized as a detachment of the superior labrum from the glenoid and the tendon of the long head of the biceps.

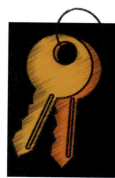

Before treating a patient's status post SLAP repair on the NPTE, it is crucial to understand the direction of instability before surgery. The direction of instability is likely to be anterior but can also be posterior.

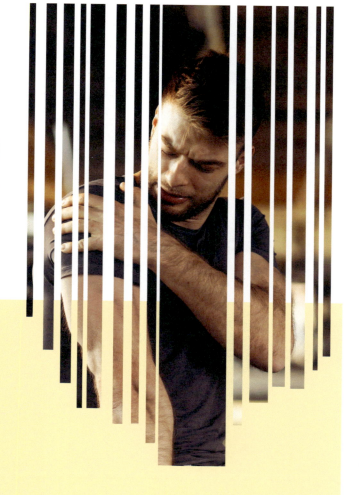

MAJOR POST-OP REHAB NOTES
- SLAP tear repairs, where the biceps tendon is detached, should be progressed more cautiously than when the biceps are intact.
- Shoulder elevation PROM is limited to 30 degrees per week (90 degrees by 3 to 4 weeks).
- Internal Rotation (IR) and External Rotation (ER) should only be performed passively or assisted.
  - Weeks 1 – 2: 0 – 15 degrees of ER and 0 – 45 degrees of IR
  - Weeks 3 – 4: 15 – 30 degrees of ER and 0 – 60 degrees of IR

MAXIMUM PROTECTION PHASE (0-6 WEEKS)

GOALS

- Reduce pain & inflammation to a minimal level.
- Protect repaired structures.
- Minimize the negative consequences of immobilization.
- Prevent reflex inhibition and disuse atrophy.

TOP 2 SPECIFIC ACTIVITIES TO AVOID

(1) For six weeks, avoid active elbow flexion/supination (active biceps contraction).
(2) Avoid shoulder extension combined with elbow extension for six weeks.

> **SPECIAL CLINICAL NOTES**
> It is essential in this phase to use modalities to reduce pain and swelling while incorporating exercises and education to improve posture. You can educate the patient about non-weighted pendulums, but they should avoid activities that involve active ROM of the affected shoulder. Gentle sub-max isometrics, called muscle setting, can often be performed with the glenohumeral musculature within the first week.

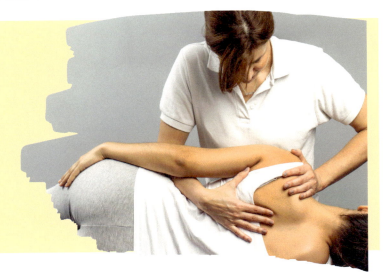

MODERATE PROTECTION PHASE (6-12 WEEKS)[32]

GOALS

- Achieve full AROM by 12 weeks.
- Increase strength and endurance required for functional activities.

TOP 4 SPECIFIC ACTIVITIES TO AVOID

(1) Avoid resisted biceps contraction for 8 – 12 weeks.
(2) Avoid abduction combined with maximal external rotation for 12+ weeks.
(3) After anterior stabilization, avoid initiating dynamic strengthening of the internal rotation from a position of full external rotation.
(4) After anterior stabilization, avoid strengthening the shoulder extensors from a shoulder extension position beyond the frontal plane.

> **SPECIAL CLINICAL NOTES**
> The primary goal of the moderate protection phase is to restore full mobility while increasing stability through dynamic strength training. Alternating isometrics, a PNF technique, is a typical entry-level exercise to begin stability training. However, clinicians recommend progressing toward dynamic resistance exercises focusing on both concentric and eccentric motion in mid-range.

"I CAN DO ALL THINGS THROUGH CHRIST WHO STRENGTHENS ME."

PHILIPPIANS 4:13

CHAPTER 25

SLIPPED CAPITAL FEMORAL EPIPHYSIS

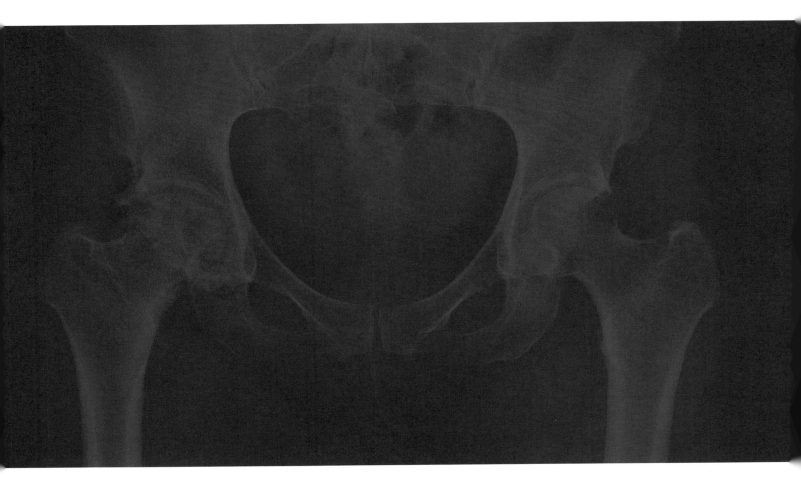

LEGG CALVE PERTHES DISEASE VS SLIPPED CAPITAL FEMORAL EPIPHYSIS[33]

	LEGG CALVE PERTHES DISEASE	SLIPPED CAPITAL FEMORAL EPIPHYSIS
PATHOPHYSIOLOGY	Avascular Necrosis	Weak femoral epiphyseal growth plates with excessive mechanical stress.
ANATOMY INVOLVED	Femoral Head	Femoral neck/Femoral epiphyseal growth plate
TRAUMATIC OR ATRAUMATIC	Insidious Onset, Atraumatic	Sudden Onset, Traumatic
AGE OF ONSET	3 – 12	12 – 15
GENDER	Male Dominant	Male Dominant
PATIENT CHARACTERISTICS	Short Stature	Overweight/Obese
LATERALITY	Primarily Unilateral	Primarily Unilateral
GAIT DEVIATIONS	Psoatic Limp or Trendelenburg	Lurch Gait or Trendelenburg
CAPSULAR PATTERN	Absent	Present
PROGNOSIS	Progression of the disease lasts 2 – 5 years. Patients often recover with conservative treatment.	Later onset yields a worse prognosis, and most patients will require surgery.
TREATMENT GOALS	Conservative treatment focused on mobility, positioning, weight-bearing, and gait training.	Immobilization, non-weight-bearing, splinting, and surgery

"TIME IS YOUR MOST PRECIOUS RESOURCE, AND PROCRASTINATION CREATES THE WORST KIND OF DEBT... PROCRASTINATION STEALS TIME & ENERGY FROM TOMORROW."

–COACH K

CHAPTER 26

SPONDYLOLISTHESIS

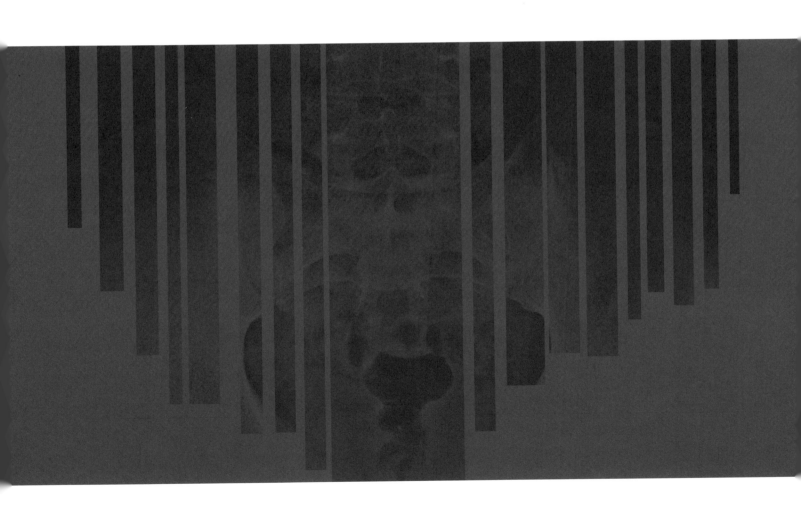

SECTION I

SPONDYLOLISTHESIS[34]

Spondylolisthesis is a forward displacement of one vertebra over another that occurs in the caudal segments of the spine.

- Anterolisthesis and retrolisthesis refer to a forward and backward displacement of one vertebra on another.
- Spondylolisthesis is most likely to occur at spinal segments L4-L5 and L5-S1.

PATHOPHYSIOLOGY

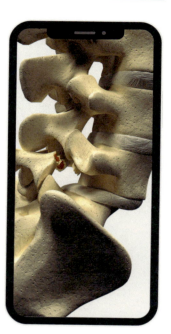

The pars interarticularis is a small segment of bone that joins the superior and inferior facets and the lamina and pedicle.

A fracture or non-union of bone in this region bilaterally creates marked instability and characteristic vertebral slippage.

DIAGNOSTIC IMAGING & SCALING

Plain Radiographic Imaging (X-Ray)

- The bilateral posterior oblique views allow for visualization of the posterior lumbar elements and pars interarticularis.
- The presentation of a non-unified pars interarticularis (i.e., decapitated Scottie dog) bilaterally is consistent with spondylolisthesis.
- Bilateral lateral views allow for visualization of the spondylolisthesis to determine severity (i.e., slippage). The Meyerding scale classifies the degree of slippage.

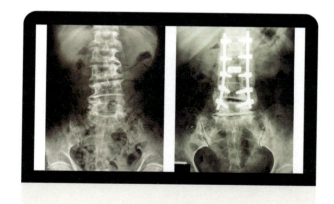

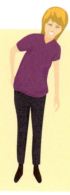

MEYERDING SCALE
GRADE 1: <25% SLIP
GRADE 2: 25-49% SLIP
GRADE 3: 50-74% SLIP
GRADE 4: 75-99% SLIP
GRADE 5: 100+% SLIP

CHAPTER 26

STEP OFF DEFORMITY

The spondylolisthesis step deformity, also called "step off sign," is a palpable anterior displacement of a spinous process relative to the level below.

In standing, the therapist runs a finger up or down the lumbar spine in search of a spinous process that is anteriorly displaced relative to the level immediately below.

When running your finger up the spinous processes, if you feel L4 anteriorly displaced relative to L5, this is called an L5-S1 spondylolisthesis.

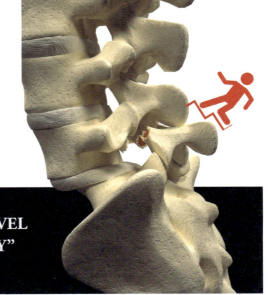

> "THE LEVEL OF THE SLIP IS ONE LEVEL BELOW THE STEP-OFF DEFORMITY"

EXTRA PRACTICE

When running your finger up the spinous processes, if you feel L3 anteriorly displaced relative to L4, this is called an L4-L5 spondylolisthesis.

When running your finger up the spinous processes, if you feel L2 anteriorly displaced relative to L3, this is called an L3-L4 spondylolisthesis.

"PUSH YOURSELF BECAUSE NO ONE IS GOING TO DO IT FOR YOU."

—COACH K

CHAPTER 27

THUMB MECHANICS

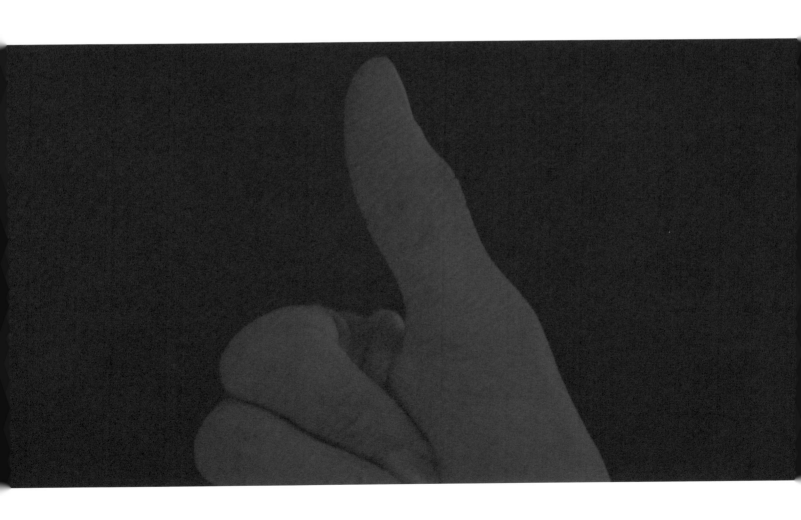

1ST CMC JOINT BIOMECHANICS

> **NPTE Special Note**
> The 1st carpometacarpal (CMC) joint comprises two bones that articulate with each other: the trapezium and the 1st metacarpal.

The 1st CMC joint is known as a saddle joint because, in one plane, the joint is convex on concave, while in another plane, the joint is concave on convex.

MASTERING THE UNI-PLANAR MOTIONS OF THE THUMB[35]		
OSTEOKINEMATIC MOTION	Flexion/Extension	Abduction/Adduction
PLANE OF MOTION	Frontal Plane	Sagittal plane
JOINT GEOMETRY	Concave on Convex	Convex on Concave
ARTHROKINEMATIC MOTION	Roll and glide in the same direction	Roll and glide in opposite directions.
ARTHROKINEMATIC EXAMPLE	For flexion, medial (ulnar roll) and medial glide.	**Abduction** • Volar (palmar roll) and the dorsal glide. **Adduction** • Dorsal (posterior roll) & volar (palmar) glide.

"SUCCESS DOESN'T COME FROM WHAT YOU DO OCCASIONALLY; IT COMES FROM WHAT YOU DO CONSISTENTLY."

–MARIE FORLEO

CHAPTER 28

TMJ BASICS

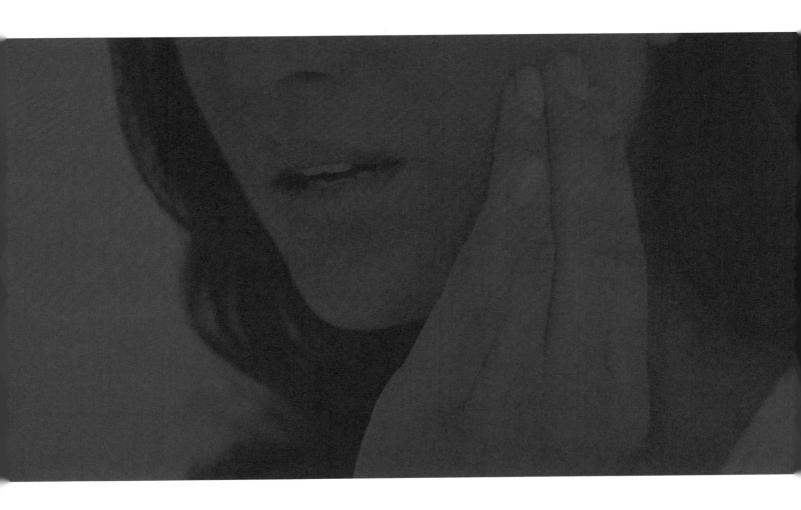

SECTION 1

TMJ BASICS REVIEW[36]

Resting Position: Mouth slightly open, lips touching, teeth not in contact.

Closed Packed Position: Teeth tightly clenched.

Capsular Pattern: Limited mouth opening.

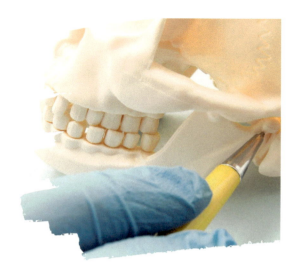

NPTE NORMAL RANGE OF MOTION

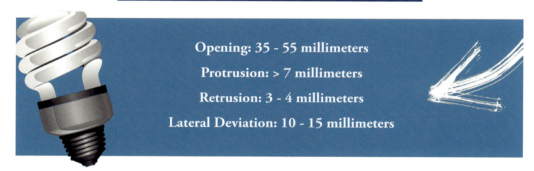

Opening: 35 - 55 millimeters

Protrusion: > 7 millimeters

Retrusion: 3 - 4 millimeters

Lateral Deviation: 10 - 15 millimeters

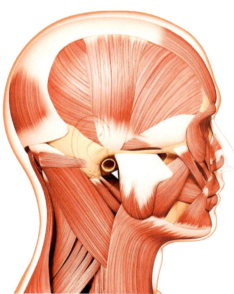

JAW OPENING MUSCULATURE

- Lateral Pterygoid
- Mylohyoid
- Geniohyoid
- Digastric

JAW CLOSING MUSCULATURE

- Medial Pterygoid
- Masseter
- Temporalis

CHAPTER 28

BITE DOWN/COTTON ROLL TMJ SPECIAL TEST

Purpose
To determine the origin of the patient's jaw pain (i.e., muscular or joint-related)

Procedure
The clinician places a tongue depressor or cotton roll on one side of the patient's mouth between teeth and then asks the patient to bite down (clench) on the object.

> *PAIN REPRODUCED ON THE **SAME SIDE** OF THE COTTON ROLL
> A MUSCLE ON THE **SAME SIDE** IS CAUSING THE PAIN*
>
> *PAIN REPRODUCED ON THE **OPPOSITE SIDE** OF THE COTTON ROLL
> THE JOINT ON THE **OPPOSITE SIDE** IS CAUSING THE PAIN*

A PRINCIPLE TO REMEMBER FOR THE NPTE

Biting down on one side stresses the temporomandibular joint on the opposite side. Therefore, if a patient bites down on the right side but feels pain on the left, the patient likely has a left temporomandibular joint problem (i.e., osteoarthritis, joint inflammation, etc.)

"DON'T LIMIT YOUR CHALLENGES... CHALLENGE YOUR LIMITS."

—COACH K

CHAPTER 29

TRICKY TRANSFERS

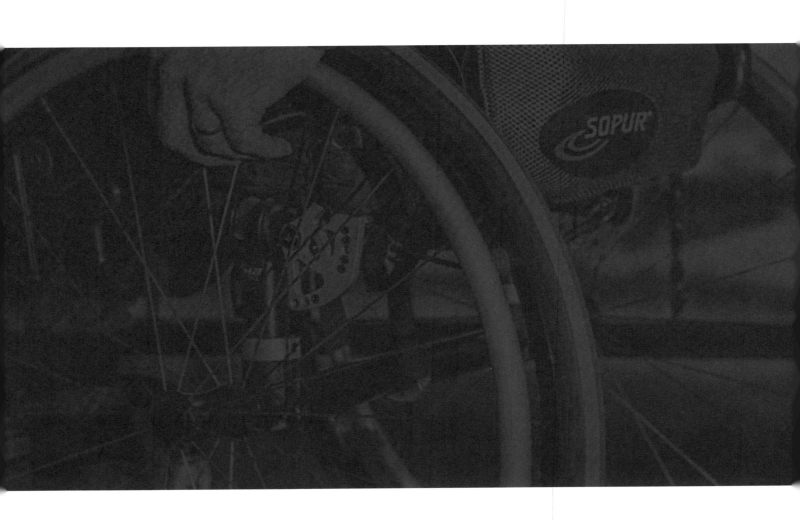

SECTION I

TOP TWO TRICKY TRANSFERS FOR THE NPTE[37]

ASCENDING & DESCENDING A CURB IN A WHEELCHAIR

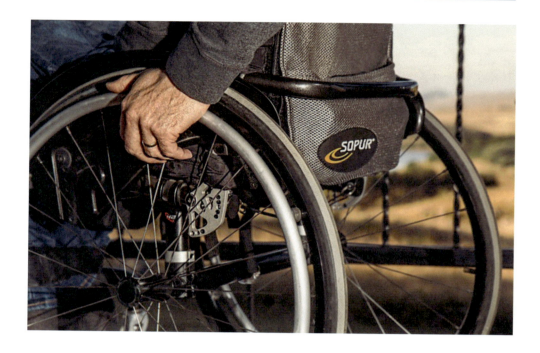

On the NPTE, descending a curb becomes tricky because individuals do it backward and forward. Let's review the most tested of the two, the backward technique.

When descending backward, back the wheelchair up to the curb's edge. Lean the body forward as you slowly reverse the rear wheels. Use your hands for friction on the rear wheels to allow the wheels to hit the lower pavement slowly. Continue to propel backward until the front casters are also on the lower pavement, and voila!

Often, one faces the curb when ascending it. The procedure includes "popping-a-wheelie" by bringing the wheelchair close to the curb. Next, the patient is instructed to pull back quickly and equally on both hand rims and then abruptly stop the rearward motion of the rear wheels by firmly grasping the hand rims.

> **Note:** Some references say that a quick push of the rear wheels anteriorly should follow the abrupt stop. When placing the front casters onto the curb, the patient can propel the rear wheels up to the curb to complete the transfer.

CHAPTER 29

ASCENDING & DESCENDING STAIRS WITH A WALKER

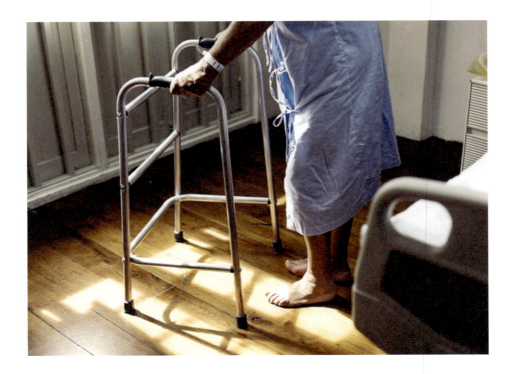

Ascending or descending stairs with a standard walker is only permitted when a patient has good balance, trunk control, and adequate extremity strength.

Ascending stairs with a standard walker and handrail

The patient places the walker on the opposite side of the handrail. The closed side of the walker is placed closest to the body. The patient places the front feet of the walker on the step above and the rear feet on the step where the patient is standing. The patient ascends with the sound limb and then lifts the affected lower extremity. The patient advances the walker to the next step.

Descending stairs with a standard walker and handrail

As with ascending, patients use the same set-up in this phase. This time, the patient places the front feet of the walker one step below and the rear feet at the level that the patient is standing. The weaker lower extremity descends first, while the strongest lower extremity controls the eccentric lowering. The walker follows, and the patient repeats the process. During this transfer, the clinician instructs the patient to grasp onto the rear hand grip or the midpoint of the horizontal bar of the walker.

CHAPTER 30

VBI TESTING

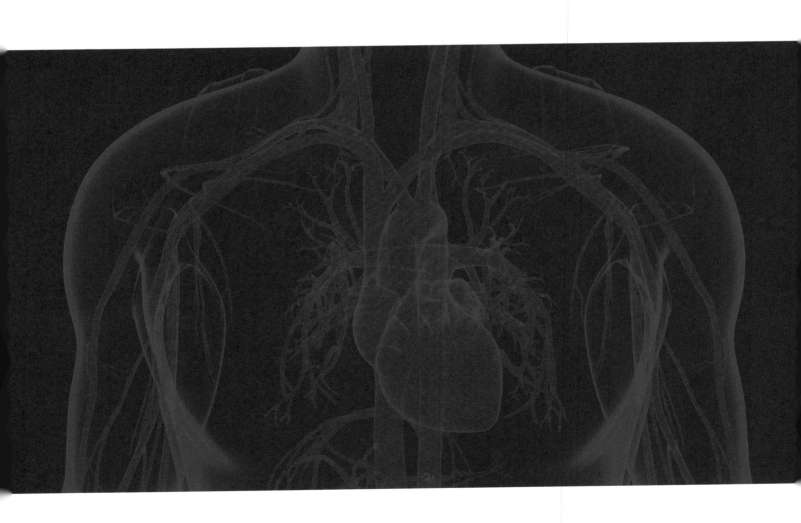

SECTION 1

VERTEBROBASILAR INSUFFICIENCY (VBI) TESTING[38]

VERTEBROBASILAR ARTERIAL SYSTEM

The vertebrobasilar arterial system is located at the back of your brain and comprises anterior and posterior vertebral arteries and a basilar artery.

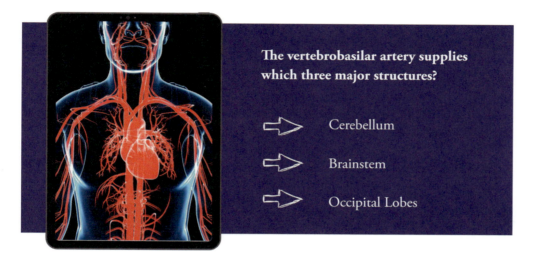

The vertebrobasilar artery supplies which three major structures?

⇨ Cerebellum

⇨ Brainstem

⇨ Occipital Lobes

VERTEBROBASILAR INSUFFICIENCY

Arterial hardening or blockage of the vertebrobasilar artery often results in poor blood flow to the posterior aspect of the brain.

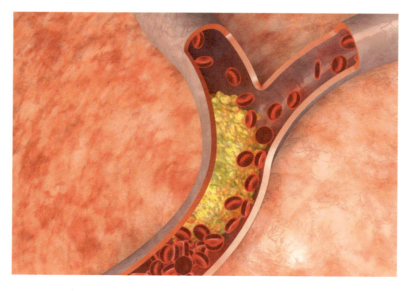

CHAPTER 30

VBI COMMON SIGNS & SYMPTOMS

"The 5 D's And The 3 N's"

D	A	N
Drop Attacks	Ataxia of gait	Nystagmus
Dysarthria		Nausea & Vomiting
Dysphagia		Numbness & Tingling
Diplopia		
Dizziness		

VBI TESTING ON THE NPTE

VERTEBRAL ARTERY (QUADRANT TEST)

Procedure:
- With the patient supine, the examiner passively extends the patient's head/neck while side bending. Once the examiner achieves this movement, the examiner rotates the patient's head/neck to the same side. The examiner holds this position for 30 seconds.

Positive Test:
- Reproduction of patient's symptoms (if this occurs, the contralateral artery is impaired).

VERTEBRAL ARTERY TESTING REMINDERS

Cervical Rotation Tests:
- Contralateral Vertebral Artery

Flexion + Rotation Tests:
- Both Vertebral Arteries

Extension + Rotation Tests:
- Contralateral Vertebral Artery

Side-bending Only:
- Ipsilateral Vertebral Artery (but minimally)

"DO YOUR BEST UNTIL YOU KNOW BETTER. THEN WHEN YOU KNOW BETTER DO BETTER"

—MAYA ANGELOU

CHAPTER 31

TYPES OF PAIN

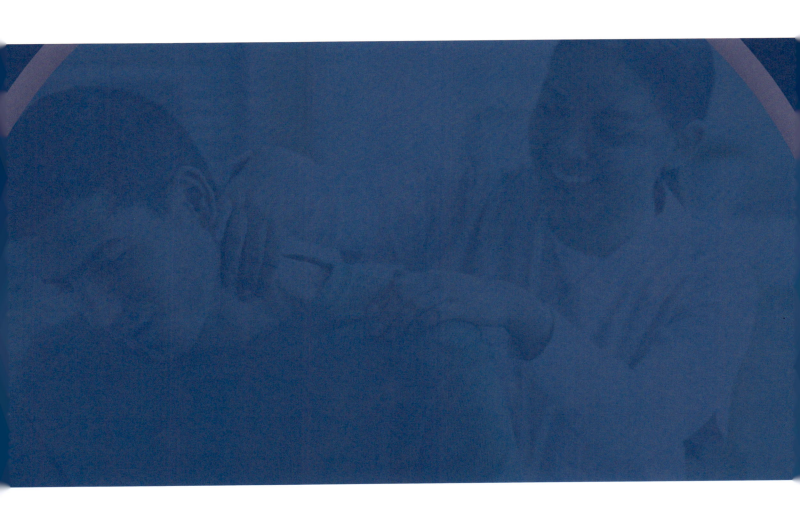

SECTION I

TYPES OF PAIN TO KNOW FOR THE NPTE[39,40,41]

ACHY PAIN

Definition:

A discomfort that is persistent but not typically intense; often associated with muscle soreness or stiffness.

Characteristics:

Continuous discomfort, dull, often spread over an area.

Examples:

a. Delayed Onset Muscle Soreness
b. Headache
c. Bone Bruises

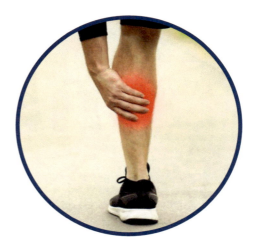

DULL PAIN

Definition:

Often, clinicians describe pain that is not sharp or intense as a mild ache or heavy feeling.

Characteristics:

Muted, not severe, poorly localized

Examples:

a. Osteoarthritis
b. Muscle soreness
c. Headache

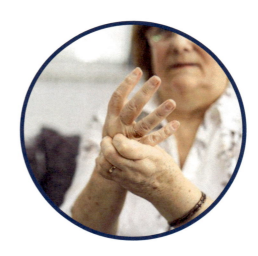

RAW PAIN

Definition:

Pain that feels like the skin or tissue is chafed or overly tender.

Characteristics:

Sore, tender, inflamed sensation.

Examples:

    a. Dry Skin
    b. Irritated Skin
    c. Psoriasis

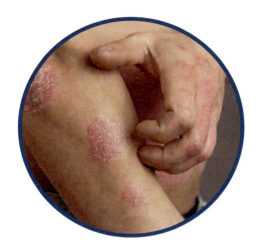

THROBBING PAIN

Definition:

Pain with a pulsating quality, often in sync with the heartbeat.

Characteristics:

Pulsing, rhythmic, can be intense.

Examples:

    a. Myocardial infarction
    b. Angina
    c. Congestive Heart Failure
    d. Aortic Aneurysm

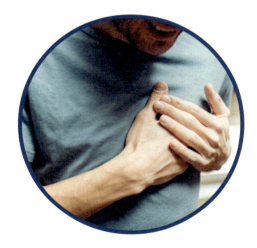

SHARP PAIN

Definition:

Often, clinicians describe pain that is intense and sudden onset as stabbing.

Characteristics:

Severe, sudden, well-localized.

Examples:

    a. Kidney stones
    b. Lacerations
    c. Appendicitis
    d. Fracture

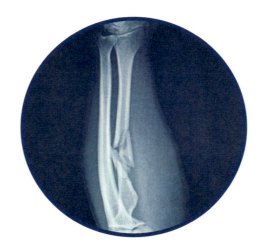

BURNING PAIN

Definition:

Pain with a scalding quality is often associated with nerve injury.

Characteristics:

Hot, stinging, sometimes accompanied by tingling.

Examples:

    a. Herpes Zoster
    b. Nerve Compression
    c. Sciatica

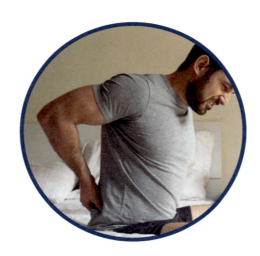

INCREDIBLE OFFER OPPORTUNITY

Are you ready to ace the NPTE and kickstart your career as a Physical Therapist? Join over 20,000 Physical Therapy graduates who have trusted Coach K's NPTE review courses and coaching programs to guide them to success.

Under Coach K's expert guidance, you'll discover the proven formula for answering every type of NPTE question with confidence. No need to spend endless hours studying—Coach K's program is designed to make your prep efficient and effective.

Don't miss out! Limited spots are available, so act fast and scan the QR code below for more information and secure your spot in this all-inclusive program.

Your dream PT career is just one step away!

CHAPTER 32

DISTINGUISHING PAIN

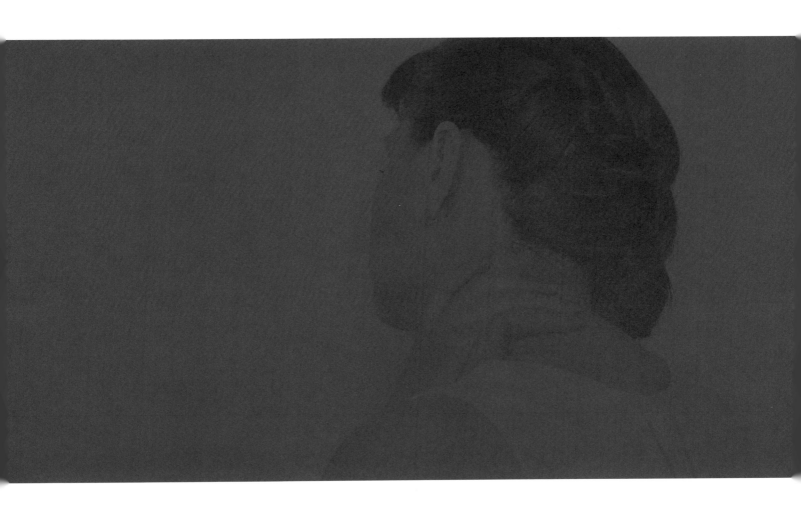

SECTION I

MYOFASCIAL PAIN SYNDROME VS FIBROMYALGIA[42,43]

MYOFASCIAL PAIN SYNDROME (MPS)

Clinicians characterize Myofascial pain syndrome as localized muscle pain triggered by discrete, irritable points in taut bands of skeletal muscle, known as trigger points.

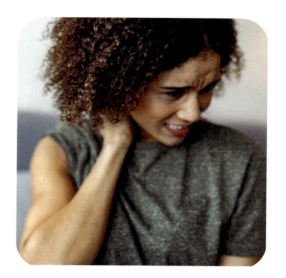

SYMPTOMS

- Localized muscle pain
- Decreased range of motion (ROM)
- Trigger points affecting a single muscle group or muscle
- Sleep disturbances due to pain
- Symptoms worsen with activity or stress

PHYSICAL EXAM

- Palpable taut bands of muscle fibers
- Reproduction of pain symptoms with palpation of trigger points

FIBROMYALGIA (FM)

A widespread pain condition involving the musculoskeletal system, often associated with fatigue and tenderness in specific areas.

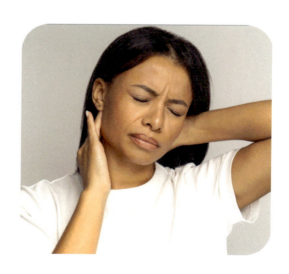

SYMPTOMS

- Widespread Muscle and Joint Pain
  - Both sides of the body, above and below the waist
- Chronic Fatigue
  - Even after long periods of sleep/rest
- Cognitive Difficulties
  - *"Fibro Fog"* – problems with memory, concentration
- Mood Disturbances
  - Depression, anxiety
- Other Symptoms
  - Headaches, irritable bowel syndrome, sleep disorders, morning stiffness

PHYSICAL EXAM
- Widespread pain that lasts for at least three months
- Presence of 11 out of 18 specific tender points
    - o Less emphasized in newer diagnostic criteria

QUICK MNEMONICS

MYOFASCIAL PAIN SYNDROME (MPS)

"L.A.M.P."

Localized Pain: Usually, the pain remains localized to a particular area.

Activity/Stress: Symptoms often worsen with activity or stress.

Muscle Knots: Tense muscle fibers often felt under the skin.

Palpable Trigger Points: Painful spots in the muscle that produce more pain when pressed.

FIBROMYALGIA (FM)

"F.A.T.I.G.U.E.D."

Fibro Fog: Cognitive difficulties, such as memory and focus issues.

All Over Pain: Widespread musculoskeletal pain.

Tiredness: Chronic fatigue.

Irritable Mood: Depression, anxiety.

Gastrointestinal Distress:

Unrefreshed Sleep: Even after a long sleep or rest, fatigue persists.

Exercise Difficulty: Physical activity can exacerbate symptoms.

Discomfort from Pressure: Pain from 11 out of 18 specific tender points on the body.

SECTION I REFERENCES

1. Bella J May, Margery A Lockard. Prosthetics & Orthotics in Clinical Practice, A Case Study Approach, pg. 261
2. Bella J May, Margery A Lockard. Prosthetics & Orthotics in Clinical Practice, A Case Study Approach, pg. 210-11
3. Bella J May, Margery A Lockard. Prosthetics & Orthotics in Clinical Practice, A Case Study Approach, pg. 213
4. Fairchild, S. L., In O'Shea, R. K., & In Washington, R. D. (2018). Pierson and Fairchild's principles & techniques of patient care.
5. Wainner RS, Irrgang JJ, Boninger ML, Delitto A, Allison S. Reliability and diagnostic accuracy of the clinical examination and patient self-report measures for cervical radiculopathy. Spine 2003;28(1):52-62.
6. Wainner R, Fritz J, Irrgang J, Delitto A, Allison S, Boninger M. Development of a Clinical Prediction Rule for the Diagnosis of Carpal Tunnel Syndrome. Arch Phys Med 2005; 86: 609-618
7. Flynn T, Fritz J, Whitman J, et al. A clinical prediction rule for classifying patients with low back pain who demonstrate short-term improvement with spinal manipulation. Spine. 2002;27(24):2835-2843.
8. Stiell IG, McKnight RD, Greenberg GH, McDowell I, Nair RC, Wells GA, Johns C, Worthington JR. Implementation of the Ottawa Ankle Rules. JAMA 1994;271:827-32.
9. Stiell IG, McKnight RD, Greenberg GH, McDowell I, Nair RC, Wells GA, Johns C, Worthington JR. Implementation of the Ottawa Ankle Rules. JAMA 1994;271:827-32.
10. Palisano, R. J., In Orlin, M. N., & In Schreiber, J. (2017). Campbell's physical therapy for children.
11. Magee, D. J. (2008). Orthopedic physical assessment. St. Louis, Mo: Saunders Elsevier.
12. Magee, D. J. (2008). Orthopedic physical assessment. St. Louis, Mo: Saunders Elsevier.
13. https://www.ncbi.nlm.nih.gov/pmc/articles/PMC3435916/
14. Neumann, Donald A. Kinesiology of the Musculoskeletal System: Foundations for Physical Rehabilitation. St. Louis: Mosby, 2002.
15. Neumann, Donald. Kinesiology of the Musculoskeletal System; Foundations For Rehabilitation. 2nd edition. 665-670
16. Goodman, C. C., & Fuller, K. S. (2015). Pathology: Implications for the physical therapist. St. Louis, Mo: Saunders/Elsevier. pg 1344 -1346
16. Magee, David J. Orthopedic Physical Assessment. St. Louis, Mo: Saunders Elsevier, 2008.
17. Neumann, Donald A. Kinesiology Of the Musculoskeletal System: Foundations for Physical Rehabilitation. St. Louis: Mosby, 2002.
18. 1. Saunders HD. Lumbar traction*. J Orthop Sports Phys Ther. 1979; 1(1): 36-45. (LEVEL 1A) 2. Kishner C, Colby LA. Therapeutic Exercise. 5th Ed; pp 427-28, 450.
19. (1) Kishner, C., Colby, L. Therapeutic Exercise. 5th edition. Pg 688-690 (2) Magee, D. Or- thopedic Physical Assessment. 6th edition. Chapter 12. (3) Neumann, D. Kinesiology of the Musculoskeletal System. 3rd Edition. pg 539-547

20 Olson, Kenneth. (2015). Manual Physical Therapy of the Spine. St. Louis, MO. Saunders Neumann, Donald A. Kinesiology Of the Musculoskeletal System: Foundations for Physical Rehabilitation. St. Louis: Mosby, 2002.

21 McKinnis, L. N. (2014). Fundamentals of musculoskeletal imaging.

22 McKinnis, L. N. (2014). Fundamentals of musculoskeletal imaging.

23 Magee, David J. Orthopedic Physical Assessment. St. Louis, Mo: Saunders Elsevier, 2008.

24 Bella, M., Lockard, M. Prosthetics & Orthotics in Clinical Practice, A Case Study Approach. 2011. Pg 121-125.

25 Bella, M., Lockard, M. Prosthetics & Orthotics in Clinical Practice, A Case Study Approach. 2011. Pg 121-125.

26 Bella, M., Lockard, M. Prosthetics & Orthotics in Clinical Practice, A Case Study Approach. 2011. Pg 121- 125.

27 Neumann, Donald A. (©2010) Kinesiology of the musculoskeletal system: foundations for rehabilitation St. Louis, Mo.: Mosby/Elsevier,

28 Goodman, C. C., & Snyder, T. K. (2013). Differential Diagnosis for Physical Therapists: Screening for Referral. London: Elsevier Health Sciences.

29 Magee, D. J. (2008). Orthopedic physical assessment. St. Louis, Mo: Saunders Elsevier.

30 Magee, D.J. (2008). Orthopedic physical assessment. St. Louis, MO: Saunders Elsevier

31 Kisner, C., & Colby, L. A. (1996) Therapeutic Exercise: Foundations and Techniques. Philadelphia: F.A. Davis

32 Kisner, C., & Colby, L. A. (1996) Therapeutic Exercise: Foundations and Techniques. Philadelphia: F.A. Davis

33 Magee, D. J. (2008). Orthopedic physical assessment. St. Louis, Mo: Saunders Elsevier. Goodman, C. C., & Fuller, K. S. (2009). Pathology: Implications for the physical therapist. St. Louis, Mo: Saunders/Elsevier.

34 Magee, David J. Orthopedic Physical Assessment. St. Louis, Mo: Saunders Elsevier, 2008.

35 Neumann, Donald A. Kinesiology Of the Musculoskeletal System: Foundations for Physical Rehabilitation. St. Louis: Mosby, 2002.

36 Magee, David J. Orthopedic Physical Assessment. St. Louis, Mo: Saunders Elsevier, 2008.

37 Fairchild, SL. Pierson and Fairchild's Principles and Techniques of Patient Care. 2013. 5th edition

38 Magee, D. J., & Magee, D. J. (2014). Orthopedic physical assessment.

39 "Differential Diagnosis for Physical Therapists: Screening for Referral" by Catherine C. Goodman and Teresa E. Kelly

40 "Physical Rehabilitation" by Susan B. O'Sullivan, Thomas J. Schmitz, George D. Fulk

41 "Pain: A Textbook for Health Professionals" by Hubert van Griensven, Jenny Strong, Anita M. Unruh

42 Goodman and Fuller's *Pathology: Implications for the Physical Therapist*

43 Travell, Simons & Simons' *Myofascial Pain and Dysfunction: The Trigger Point Manual*

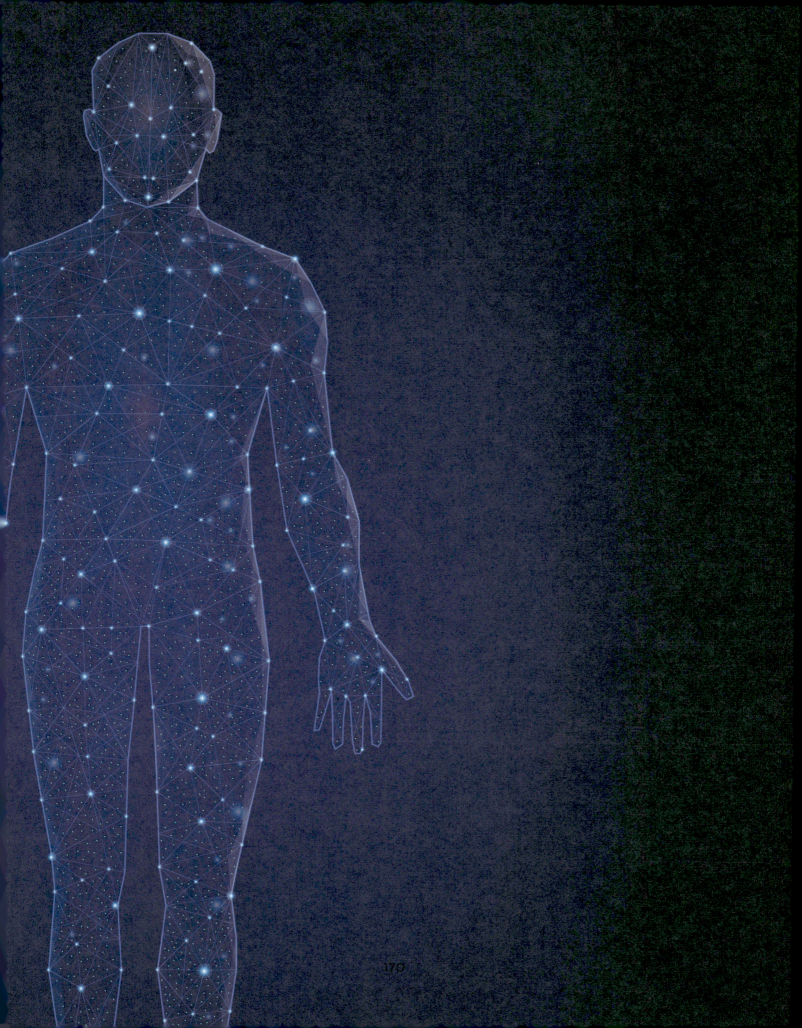

SECTION II

NEUROMUSCULAR CHEAT SHEETS

CHAPTER 33

APHASIA

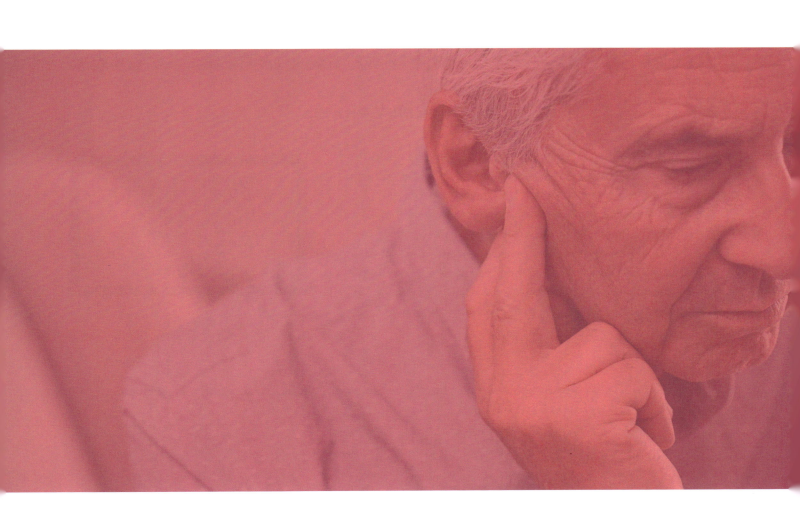

SECTION 11

TYPES OF APHASIA TO KNOW

BROCA'S APHASIA

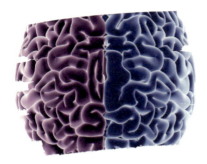

- A middle cerebral artery stroke (MCA) typically causes Broca's aphasia, with the lesion located in the premotor area of the left frontal lobe.
- Patients with Broca's aphasia display a slowed and hesitant speech pattern and limited vocabulary.
- Patients present with difficulty properly arranging words into well-formed sentences.

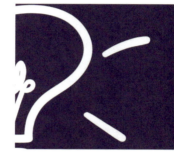

"**B.E.N.** has Broca's"
- **B**roca's Aphasia can also be called **E**xpressive or **N**on-fluent aphasia on the NPTE.
- The saying is an easy way to remember these interchangeable names.
- **B**roca's, **E**xpressive, **N**on-fluent

WERNICKE'S APHASIA[1]

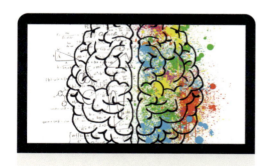

- A middle cerebral artery stroke (MCA) typically causes Wernicke's aphasia, with the lesion located in the auditory association cortex of the left lateral temporal lobe.
- In Wernicke's aphasia, speech flows smoothly with a preserved melody but often becomes incoherent.
- The patient's auditory comprehension is impaired. Thus, the patient demonstrates difficulty with comprehending spoken language and following commands. In many cases, the patient is also unable to understand written words.

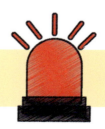

Wernicke's aphasia is also known as Receptive aphasia, Sensory aphasia, or Fluent aphasia on the NPTE.

GLOBAL APHASIA

- A middle cerebral artery stroke (MCA) typically causes Global aphasia, with the lesion in the third frontal convolution and the posterior aspect of the superior temporal gyrus.
- Global aphasia merges the characteristics of Broca's and Wernicke's aphasia, resulting in non-fluent speech and poor comprehension.
- This is the most severe form of aphasia, often indicating severe brain damage.
- Patients with global aphasia have a significantly poorer prognosis than other forms of aphasia.

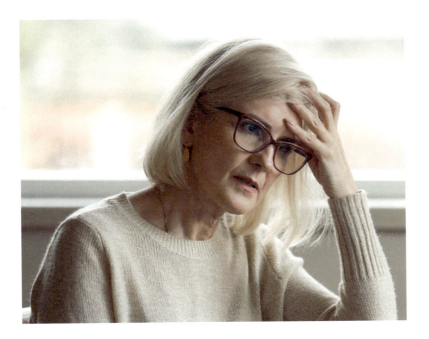

COMMON TREATMENTS

Promoting Aphasics' Communication Effectiveness (PACE)
- If your patient likes the game "Charades," they will find this therapy fun!
- The primary goal of this treatment is to improve the patient's conversational skills.
- During treatment, the patient and the clinician take turns being the message sender or receiver. The message sender gets a picture prompt and must use different communication modalities to convey the message.

Visual Action Therapy (VAT)
- Therapists most often use VAT with patients who have global aphasia.
- VAT is a non-verbal treatment that consists of 12 progressively difficult levels.
- The patient will begin tracing common objects, followed by matching objects to the tracing.
- The patient will later progress to pantomiming tasks, where gestures identify visible objects and symbolize absent objects.

> "BE WILLING TO SACRIFICE ANYTHING, BUT COMPROMISE NOTHING IN YOUR QUEST TO BE YOUR BEST."
>
> —KOBE BRYANT

CHAPTER 34

CENTRAL CORD SYNDROME DIFFERENTIAL

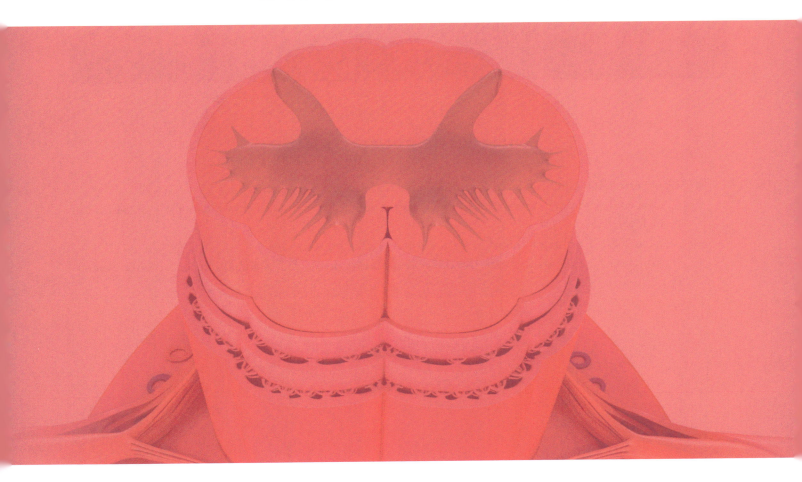

CENTRAL CORD SYNDROME[2]

WHAT ARE THE BASICS?

Central cord syndrome is the MOST COMMON type of spinal cord injury (SCI), typically due to a traumatic hyperextension of the cervical region.

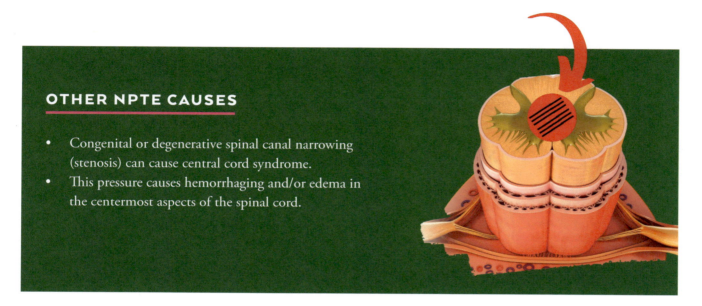

OTHER NPTE CAUSES

- Congenital or degenerative spinal canal narrowing (stenosis) can cause central cord syndrome.
- This pressure causes hemorrhaging and/or edema in the centermost aspects of the spinal cord.

WHAT'S THE PRESENTATION?

- Upper extremity motor function is impaired more than the lower extremities.
- Central cord syndrome can have impaired superficial and deep sensations below the injury level, which can be highly variable.
- This type of SCI requires minimal to no bowel and bladder impairments.
- It's common for patients to regain the ability to ambulate due to SCI's limited impact on lower extremity function.

"THIS IS THE OPPORTUNITY TO SHOW YOURSELF THAT ANYTHING IS POSSIBLE WHEN YOU WANT IT BAD ENOUGH."

–COACH K

CHAPTER 35

COMMON FEEDBACK TYPES

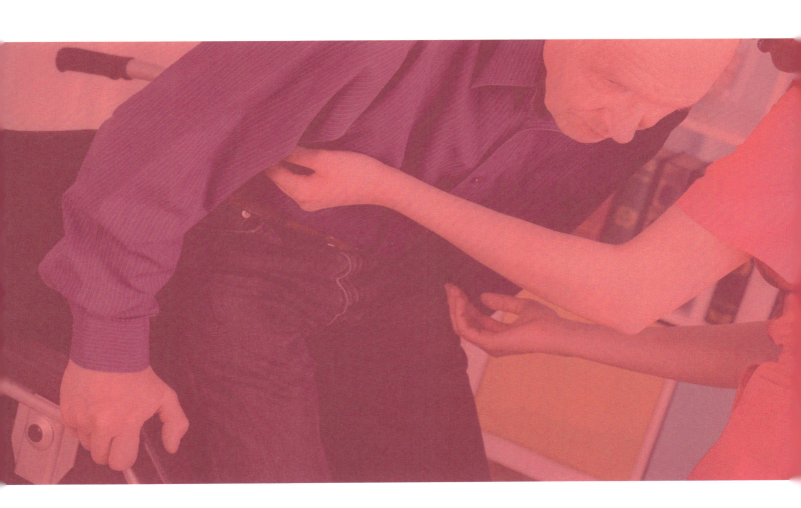

FEEDBACK TYPES

CONCURRENT FEEDBACK

Therapists present concurrent feedback to the patient during the movement, providing general information about the quality or nature of the movement, such as joint position, speed, or smoothness of motion.

> **Special NPTE Notes**
> It would be best if you used concurrent feedback when intrinsic feedback isn't easily accessible and when it connects to an active problem-solving process. Clinicians commonly see this feedback form in the associative and autonomous motor learning stages.

DELAYED FEEDBACK

Delayed feedback is any form of feedback provided after a brief delay once the movement has ended (e.g., a 3-second delay).

> **Special NPTE Notes**
> - The purpose of the delay is to provide a brief period of introspection and self-assessment. This period of self-assessment improves retention of the task.
> - Delayed feedback can be used in any motor learning stage when the focus is on improving retention.

BANDWIDTH FEEDBACK

The therapist provides this feedback form only when the patient's performance deviates from the "correct" performance.

> **Special NPTE Notes**
> - What is considered "correct performance" is always pre-determined before the start of the task. Many therapists use this type of feedback to prevent the formation of bad habits or to intervene when a patient poses a safety risk.
> - Clinicians provide this feedback form in any of the motor learning stages.

SUMMARY FEEDBACK

Summary feedback, also known as "summed feedback" or "average feedback," is feedback provided after a set number of trials (e.g., after every 2nd, 6th, or 20th trial).

> **Special NPTE Notes**
> - Summary feedback has improved skill retention while significantly delaying skill acquisition dramatically.
> - Many therapists use this form in the cognitive and associative motor learning stages.

FADED FEEDBACK

Therapists provide this form of feedback after every trial and then less frequently on subsequent blocks of trials (e.g., after every trial, then after every 3rd trial, then after every 5th trial, etc.).

> **Special NPTE Notes**
> - Faded feedback is often used in the early stages of motor learning to transition from acquisition to retention-based education.
> - aded feedback allows for continued feedback while allowing the patient to self-assess and actively solve problems.

"STOP ACTING LIKE YOU WEREN'T BORN TO STAND OUT... CLAIM WHAT'S YOURS."

–COACH K

CHAPTER 36

CRANIAL NERVES

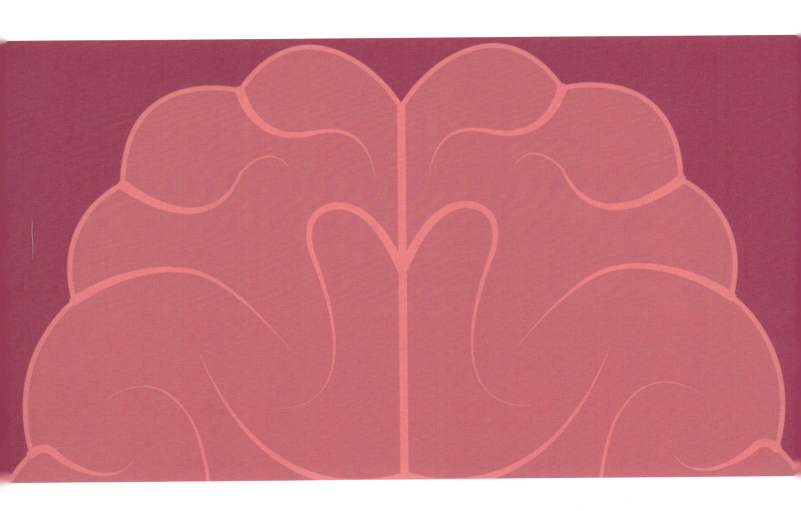

SECTION II

THE MUST-KNOW CRANIAL NERVES FOR THE NPTE

CRANIAL NERVE	FUNCTION	COMMON PATHOLOGIES	IMPORTANT TESTS
OPTIC NERVE (CN II)	Sensory Nerve: Sight/Central & Peripheral Vision	Multiple Sclerosis Middle/Posterior CVA	Snellen Visual Acuity & Confrontation
OCULOMOTOR NERVE (CN III)	Elevates Eyelids, Constricts Pupil, Turns Eye up, down and in	Multiple Sclerosis Horner's Syndrome	Pupillary Reactions, H-test, Saccadic/pursuit test
TRIGEMINAL NERVE (CN V)	Sensation from the face, cornea, and anterior tongue, muscles of mastication, & dampens sound	ALS Trigeminal Neuralgia	Clench teeth/hold against resistance, Corneal Reflex, pain, and light touch sensation (forehead, cheeks, and jaw)
FACIAL NERVE (CN VII)	Taste from anterior 2/3 of the tongue, muscles of facial expression, tearing, salivation	ALS Bell's palsy Guillain-Barre	Raise eyebrows, frown, smile big, close eyes tightly, and puff out cheeks & ability to taste sweet on the anterior 2/3 of the tongue.
GLOSSOPHA-RYNGEAL (CN IX)	Taste from posterior 1/3 of the tongue, sensation from posterior tongue and oropharynx, salivation	ALS Medullary Stroke Guillain-Barre	Ability to taste sweet on posterior 1/3 of tongue, swallowing, and phonation
VAGUS NERVE (CN X)	Thoracic and abdominal viscera, muscles of larynx and pharynx, sensation from oropharynx	ALS Medullary Stroke Guillain-Barre	Swallowing & phonation, Gag reflex, Say "ah" – Uvula Deviation Test
HYPOGLOSSAL NERVE (CN XII)	Tongue movements	ALS Multiple Sclerosis	Phonation/Articulation, Tongue movement side to side, protruding tongue

"THE BAD NEWS IS...TIME FLIES. THE GOOD NEWS IS...YOU ARE THE PILOT"

—COACH K

CHAPTER 37

GROSS MOTOR FUNCTION AND CEREBRAL PALSY

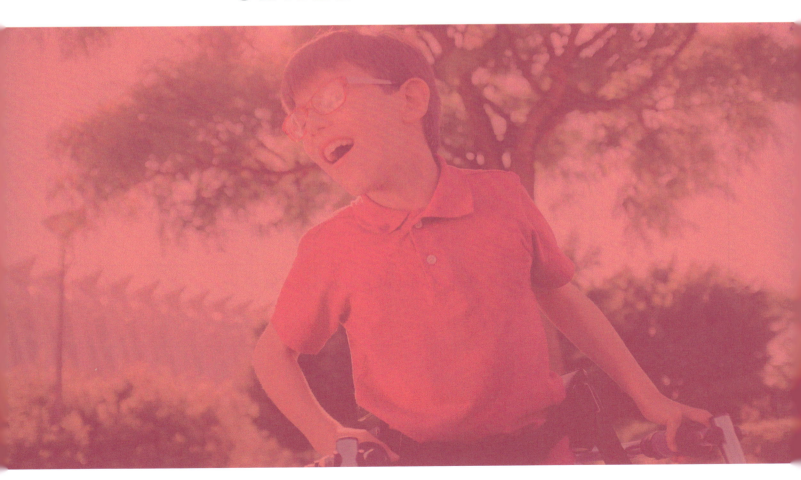

SECTION II

GROSS MOTOR FUNCTION CLASSIFICATION SCALE (GMFCS)[5]

- A 5-level standardized assessment tool for classifying a child with a motor disability (e.g., cerebral palsy).
- Clinicians base the GMFCS on "usual performance," which is what the child does regularly rather than what the child is capable of.

THE 5 LEVELS OF GMFCS

When classifying a child between the ages of 6-12, use the descriptions below:

LEVEL 1 – Walks without limitations	LEVEL 2 – Walks with limitations
Independent ambulation Climbs steps without railing. Runs & jumps. Has limited speed, balance, and coordination.	Independent ambulation in most settings. Climbs steps with railing. Requires an assistive device with environments that challenge balance. Uses wheeled mobility for long distances.
LEVEL 3 – Walks using a hand-held mobility device.	**LEVEL 4 – Self-mobility with limitations may use power-mobility.**
Walks with an assistive device in most settings. Wheeled mobility for longer distances. May climb stairs with railing and supervision.	Uses a power wheelchair or requires physical assistance for mobility in most settings. May ambulate with an assistive device and physical assistance but only short distances.
LEVEL 5 – Transported in a manual wheelchair.	
Children are transported in a manual wheelchair in all settings.	

"COMPARISON IS THE THIEF OF JOY"

—COACH K

CHAPTER 38

LATERAL MEDULLARY SYNDROME

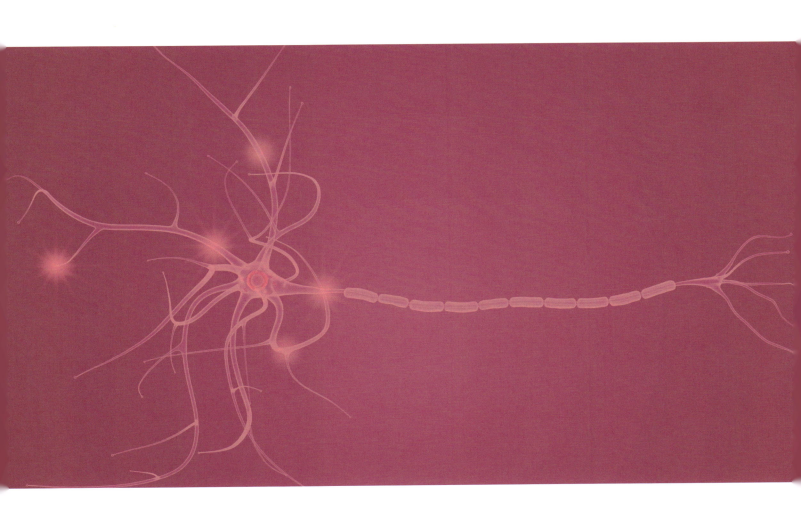

WHAT IS LATERAL MEDULLARY SYNDROME?[6]

Lateral Medullary Syndrome, also known as Wallenberg Syndrome or Posterior Inferior Cerebellar Artery (PICA) Syndrome, is a neurological condition caused by a blockage of the vertebral artery (VA) or posterior inferior cerebellar artery, which leads to infarction of the lateral medulla oblongata.

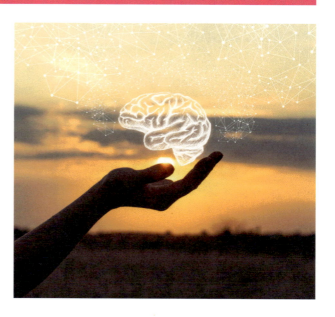

THE MEDULLA OBLONGATA

Houses 4 major cranial nerves, which can be affected by lateral medullary syndrome.
- CN IX: Glossopharyngeal
- CN X: Vagus
- CN XI: Accessory
- CN XII: Hypoglossal

DID YOU KNOW?

Cranial Nerve V, also known as the trigeminal nerve, is commonly affected, leading to characteristic pain and temperature loss on the ipsilateral face.

SIGNS AND SYMPTOMS MNEMONIC

"B.I.G. H.A.N.D.F.U.L."

Bradycardia
Ipsilateral facial sensation loss
Gag reflex diminished

Horner's Sign
Ataxia
Nystagmus
Double vision (Diplopia)
Faulty speech (Dysphonia)
Unable to swallow (Dysphagia)
Loss of contralateral limb sensation

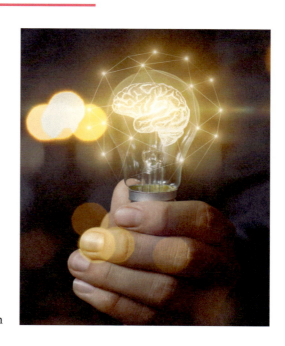

"DON'T ASPIRE TO MAKE A LIVING. ASPIRE TO MAKE A DIFFERENCE."

—DENZEL WASHINGTON

CHAPTER 39

MYASTHENIA GRAVIS

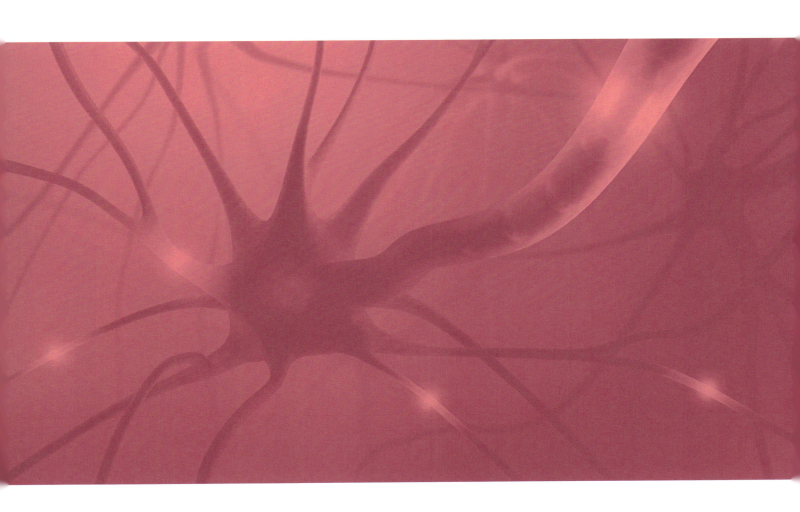

MYASTHENIA GRAVIS (MG)[7]

- An autoimmune disorder whose action occurs at the site of the neuromuscular junction and motor endplate.
- MG is commonly confused with Multiple Sclerosis because of the frequent exacerbations of the condition with stress and overworking.
- Patients with MG experience excessive fatigue as the day progresses or with prolonged activity.
- These patients also present with a characteristic improvement in strength after rest.

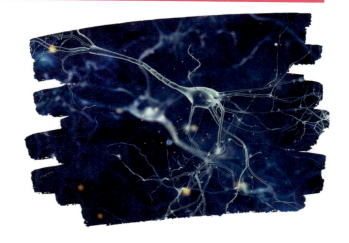

NPTE TIP

75% of people with MG have abnormalities of the thymus.

PATIENT PROFILE

- Female-dominated with a ratio of 3:2
- Females with MG are typically 20 - 30 years old.
- Males with MG are typically 50 - 60 years old.
- Patients with MG commonly have one or more of the following:
    o Hyperthyroidism
    o Thyrotoxicosis
    o Thymic tumor
    o Overactive thymic gland

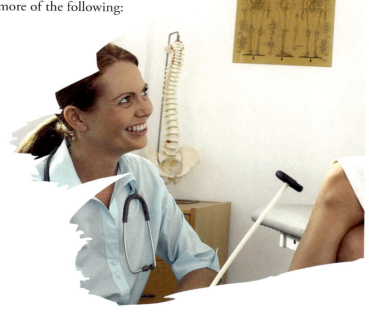

SIGNS & SYMPTOMS

- Dysarthria
- Dysphasia
- Dysphonia
- Diplopia
- Daily fluctuations in fatigue
- Proximal muscle weakness
- Ptosis & facial weakness

NPTE TIP

There are no sensory deficits with Myasthenia Gravis.

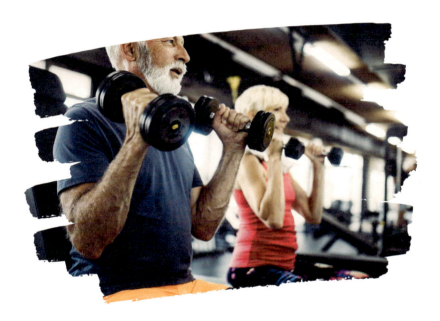

NPTE EXERCISE CONSIDERATIONS

- Avoid strenuous exercise and stress.
- Avoid prolonged exposure to hot or cold environments.
- Cautiously allow and monitor eccentric-based exercises.
- If therapists expose a patient with MG to the environments and/or activities mentioned above, they risk exacerbating the patient's symptoms.

"GOOD THINGS COME TO THOSE WHO WAIT… NOT JUST PATIENTLY, BUT IN FAITH."

–COACH K

CHAPTER 40

NEURAL TENSION TESTING

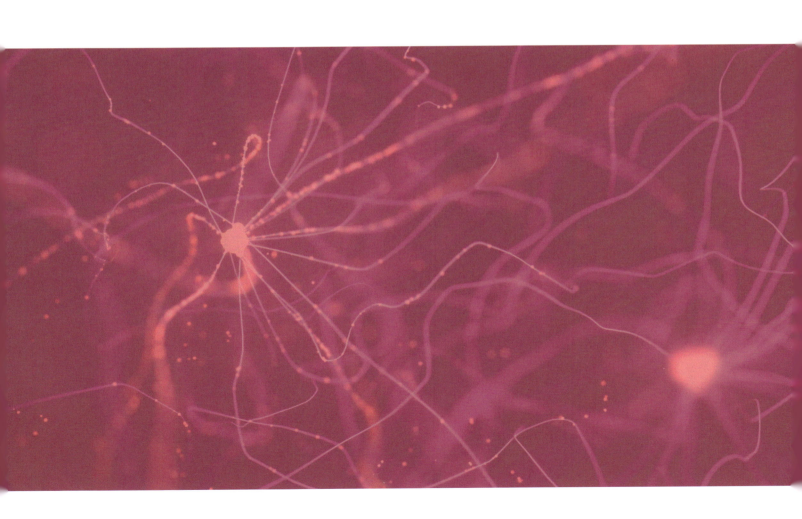

SECTION II

NERVES	NERVE TEST	PATIENT POSITION	LOWER EXTREMITY PLACEMENTS
FEMORAL NERVE	Slump	Side-Lying	Cervical, Thoracic, and Lumbar Flexion (slump) Hip Flexion (20 degrees) Knee Flexion Ankle Plantarflexion
OBTURATOR NERVE	Slump	Sitting	Cervical, Thoracic, and Lumbar Flexion (slump) Hip Abduction, Hip Flexion (90+ degrees) Knee Extension Ankle Dorsiflexion
SURAL NERVE	Straight Leg Raise (SLR)	Supine	Hip Flexion Knee Extension Ankle Dorsiflexion Foot Inversion
COMMON PERONEAL (FIBULAR) NERVE	Straight Leg Raise (SLR)	Supine	Hip Flexion & Internal Rotation Knee Extension Ankle Plantarflexion Foot Inversion
SCIATIC NERVE	Straight Leg Raise (SLR)	Supine	Hip Flexion & Adduction Knee Extension Ankle Dorsiflexion
TIBIAL NERVE	Straight Leg Raise (SLR)	Supine	Hip Flexion Knee Extension Ankle Dorsiflexion Foot Eversion Toe Extension

8

"YOU GET WHAT YOU PAY FOR… BUT MOST OF ALL, YOU GET WHAT YOU WORK FOR."

—VANESSA BOSCAN

CHAPTER 41

PARKINSONIAN GAIT INTERVENTIONS

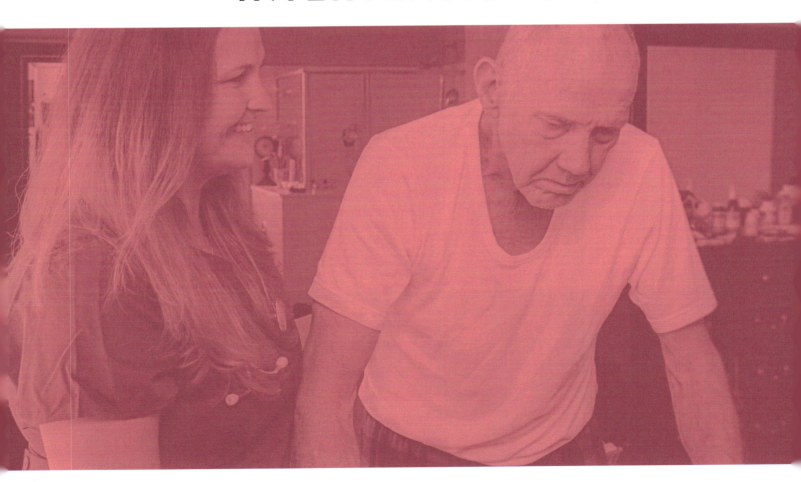

FLOOR MARKERS[9,10]

Floor markers are a visual aid to enhance attention in patients with Parkinson's disease. When someone places markers on the floor, they ask the patient to step on or over them.

Primary Uses

- Improve attention
- Improve Freezing of Gait (FOG)
- FOG Hypokinesia

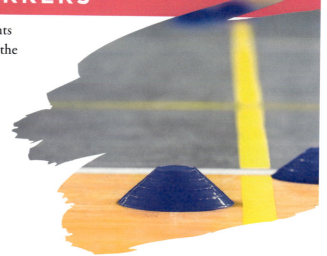

U-WALKER WITH LASER

- The U-Walker is a commonly used assistive device for patients with Parkinson's disease. The U-walker comes modifiable with a push-down braking system, elevated handles for upright posture, and a laser projection onto the floor.
- The U-Walker improves stability and upright posturing while reducing freezing of gait (FOG) and hypokinesia.

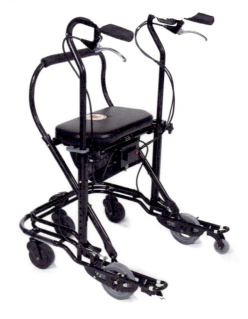

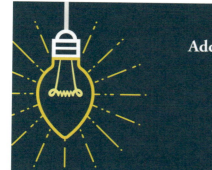

Additional visual cues that improve attention and reduce FOG

- Dropping pennies on the ground to step over
- Dropping a Kleenex
- Walking alongside the patient
- If using a cane, turn it upside down

CHAPTER 41

RHYTHMIC AUDITORY STIMULATION (METRONOME)

The metronome is a form of auditory stimulus provided to the patient to set a specific number of steps per minute (i.e., cadence).

Primary Uses

- Improve cadence
- Improve stride length
- Improve gait speed

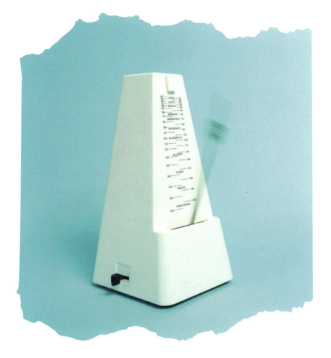

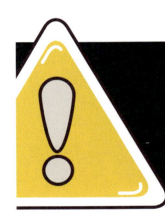

Rhythmic Auditory Stimulation is one of the most effective forms of treatment for Parkinsonian gait.

When setting the metronome, the speed should be 25% faster than the patient's current gait speed.

"IF YOU FEEL THAT YOU CAN'T DO GREAT THINGS, DO SMALL THINGS IN A GREAT WAY"

– NAPOLEAN HILL

CHAPTER 42

PNF LEAD ARM

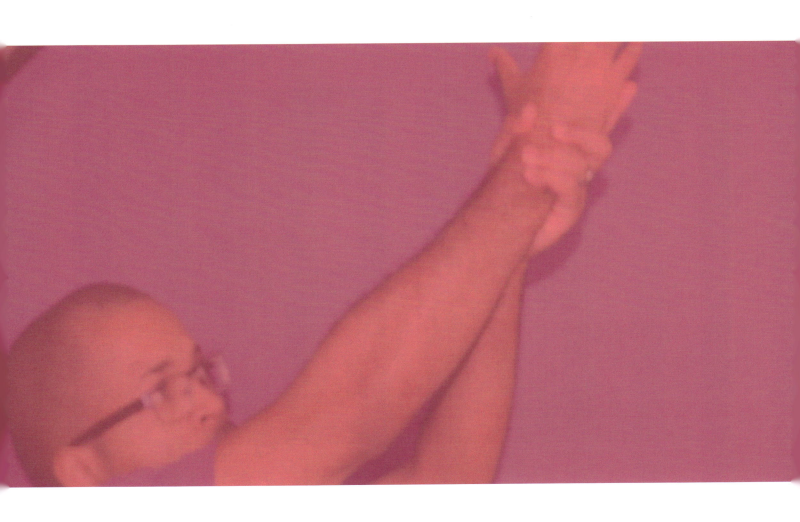

SECTION 11

MASTERING THE LEAD ARM WHEN TREATING A PATIENT WITH PNF TECHNIQUES[11]

LEAD ARM: BASIC DEFINITION

The arm that has the hand free is considered **the lead arm.**

Figure 1: the right hand is free; therefore, it is **the lead arm**

When treating your patient, the lead arm **can be either the affected or the non-affected extremity**.

Whether to use the affected or non-affected extremity as the lead arm depends on the specific PNF pattern you are trying to achieve. (e.g., D2 flexion, D1 extension, etc.)

How would you name Figure 1?
    D2 flexion pattern with the right arm leading

How would you name Figure 2?
    D1 flexion pattern with the right arm leading

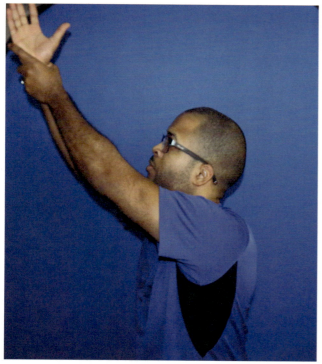 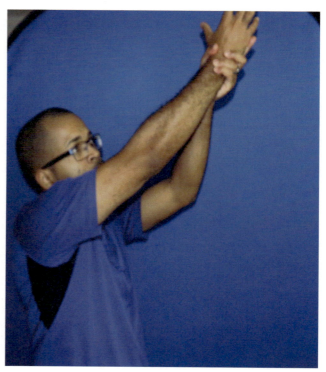

FIGURE 1 **FIGURE 2**

CHAPTER 42

If I wanted my patient to perform left upper extremity D1 flexion (reverse chop), how can I name it using the lead arm verbiage?

Left UE D1 flexion with left arm leading OR
Right UE D2 flexion with right arm leading

Both of these positions will put the left arm into D1 flexion.

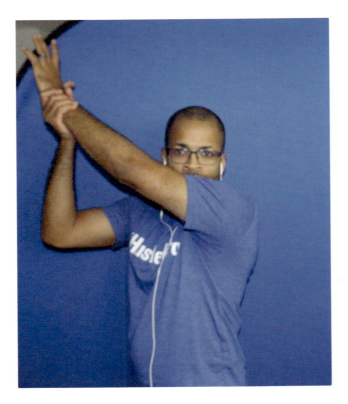

Left UE D1 flexion with left arm leading.

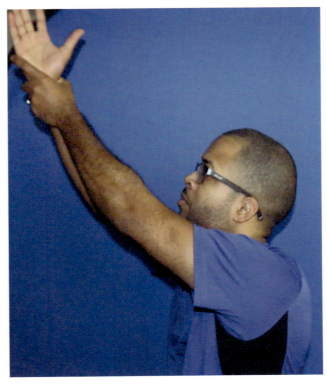

Right UE D2 flexion with right arm leading.

If I wanted my patient to perform right upper extremity D2 extension (reverse lift), how can I name it using the lead arm verbiage?

**Right UE D2 extension with right arm leading OR
Left UE D1 Extension with left arm leading**

Both of these positions will put the right arm into D2 Extension.

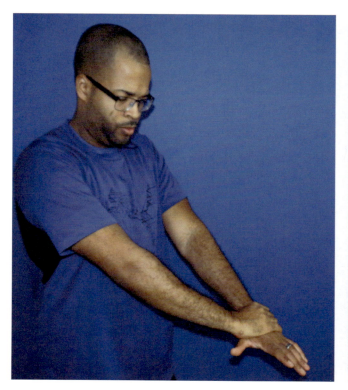

Left UE D1 flexion with left

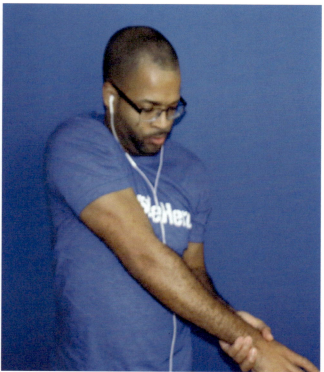

Right UE D2 flexion with right arm leading arm leading.

CHAPTER 42

MOCK NPTE-BASED QUESTION & RATIONALE

A patient with a recent middle cerebral artery (MCA) stroke presents with significant right upper extremity spasticity but can perform some motions out of synergy. The therapist would like to continue improving the patient's mobility and activation of the muscles out of synergy. Which of the following is the BEST intervention to address the current impairment?

A. Lift pattern with right arm leading

B. Bilateral PNF UE D2 Extension

C. Chop pattern with left arm leading

D. Rhythmic rotation in a side-lying position

Rationale:

The patient is in stage 4 Brunnstrom, characterized by the ability to perform some motions out of synergy. The question doesn't explicitly state a specific synergy for the upper extremity; thus, we can deduce that the patient displays dominant synergy components such as elbow flexion, shoulder adduction, and forearm pronation. We must find an intervention that focuses on bringing the patient out of synergy to assist with the progression of their mobility.

A. Lift pattern with right arm leading is correct because the patient moves into the PNF D2 flexion pattern with the affected upper extremity. This position moves the patient out of synergy. The positions included in this movement are shoulder abduction, shoulder external rotation, shoulder flexion, elbow extension, forearm supination, wrist and finger extension

B. Bilateral PNF UE D2 Extension is not an appropriate intervention because the patient lacks the voluntary capability to perform this activity alone without assistance from the therapist or the non-affected extremity. Bilateral PNF UE D2 Extension is an in-synergy motion including shoulder adduction, forearm pronation, and shoulder internal rotation.

C. Chop pattern with left arm leading is not an appropriate intervention because when the patient performs the chop pattern with the left arm leading, the patient moves into PNF D2 extension with the affected arm. This intervention is not appropriate for reasons explained in rationale B.

D. Rhythmic rotation in a side-lying position, although an excellent option for spasticity, is generally not specific to improving out-of-synergy movement with the affected upper extremity. Rhythmic rotation is a passive trunk rotation to reduce tone, spasticity, or rigidity.

CHAPTER 43

PUSHER'S SYNDROME

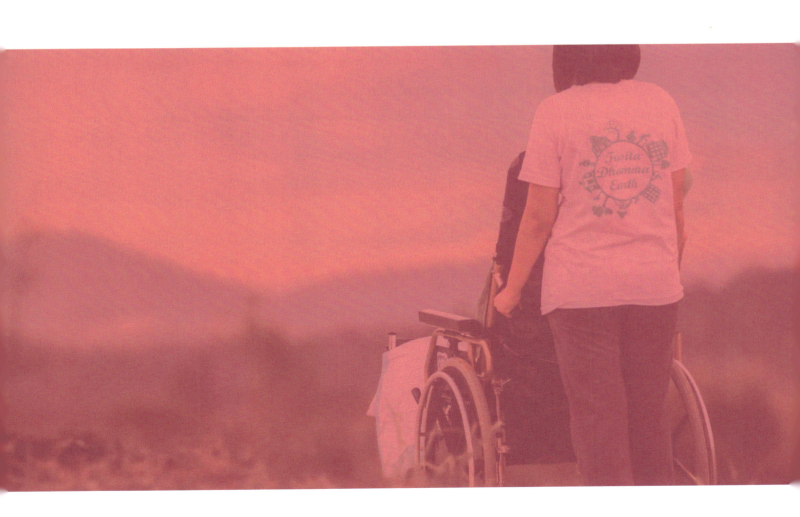

PUSHER'S SYNDROME[12]

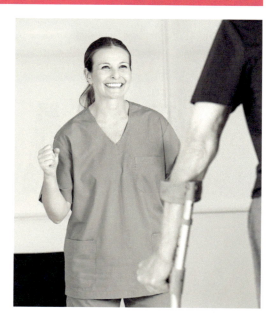

- Patients with this condition push their stronger extremities toward their weaker hemiparetic side.
- A stroke or damage to the posterolateral thalamus most often causes this condition.
- Physiologically, the patient's altered perception of their body orientation causes this behavior.
- In other words, your patient feels they're standing or sitting upright when tilted 20 degrees towards the weak side.
- Don't worry; the prognosis is good, and the brain can compensate with adequate training.
- This condition is also termed **contraversive pushing** or **ipsilateral pushing**.

TWO PROBLEMS THAT YOU SHOULD KNOW

A Significant Risk for Falls During Functional Activities

Because of their altered perception, these patients push themselves onto a weaker extremity that cannot support them. During treatment, placing a cane into the uninvolved hand or standing on the uninvolved side is often tempting. However, if not careful, the patient can use the cane to push themselves onto the weaker side, increasing the risk of falls.

They Can't Just " Stop Pushing"!

Since a patient with pusher's syndrome has an actual impairment in body orientation awareness, simple cues such as "stand up straight" are not effective. Likewise, passively pushing the patient into the correct alignment is counterproductive and may reinforce the behavior.

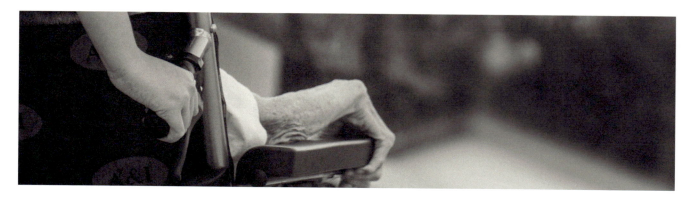

DO LIST	DON'T LIST
Use visual cues such as ground-vertical structures, vertical markings on the wall, or even the therapist's arm held upright.	Don't attempt to passively push the patient into the correct alignment, as this will increase patient frustration and reinforce patient pushing.
Allow the patient to utilize a cane (*if appropriate) in the uninvolved hand set at a lower height to encourage weight-bearing through the uninvolved side.	Don't allow the patient's sound extremities to drift into abduction and/or extension and push.
Enable the patient to realize their disturbed perception while providing ample opportunities for correct visual feedback.	Don't provide continuous solutions to orientation problems. Allow the patient to solve problems for themselves.
Ensure patient safety by utilizing strategies to guard the patient's involved side to prevent falls.	
Have the patient continuously reassess themselves to determine if they are upright by asking, "What direction are you tilted?"	
Provide consistent and quality-based feedback about where a patient is in space.	

"IF YOU WANT YOUR DREAM JOB, THEN BE PREPARED TO STOP AT NOTHING TO GET IT. "

–COACH K

CHAPTER 44

SPINA BIFIDA

SECTION II

SPINA BIFIDA IN CHILDREN[13]

Based on cognition, functional mobility and stability, and energy cost, the child with lumbar-level spina bifida requires specific orthotics or equipment, as reflected in the motor descriptions and functional outcomes below.

L1	**Quick Motor Description:** 1. Complete Trunk Function 2. Hip Flexors 2/5 or less 3. Loss of muscle function below L1	**Community Mobility:** Wheelchair Use **Household Mobility:** Walker **Orthotic Prescription:** Parapodium, RGO (coordination required), HKAFO
L2	**Quick Motor Description:** 1. Complete Trunk Function 2. Hip Flexors & Adductors 3/5 3. Quads 2/5 or less	**Community Mobility:** Wheelchair Use **Household Mobility:** Walker, Wheelchair **Orthotic Prescription:** Parapodium, RGO (coordination required), HKAFO, KAFO
L3	**Quick Motor Description:** 1. Complete Trunk Function 2. Hip Flexors & Adductors >3/5 3. Quads 3/5	**Community Mobility:** Wheelchair Use **Household Mobility:** Walker, Crutches, Wheelchair **Orthotic Prescription:** HKAFO & KAFO (if knee extensor MMT < 3/5)
L4	**Quick Motor Description:** 1. Complete Trunk/Hip/Knee Function 2. Ankle Dorsiflexors 3/5 3. Medial Knee flexors 3/5	**Community Mobility:** Walker, Cane, Crutches **Household Mobility:** May need no support **Orthotic Prescription:** AFO
L5	**Quick Motor Description:** 1. Complete Trunk/Hip/Knee Function 2. Ankle dorsiflexion is good 3. Hip abductors 2/5 4. Ankle inversion 3/5	**Community Mobility:** Walker, Cane, Crutches **Household Mobility:** May not need support **Orthotic Prescription:** AFO

CHAPTER 45

STAGES OF MOTOR LEARNING

SECTION II

STAGES OF MOTOR LEARNING TREATMENT[14]

For the NPTE, we recommend that every student thoroughly understands the three stages of motor learning and knows which types of practice and feedback to provide in each stage.

This cheat sheet will provide you with general information regarding feedback and practice types to provide in each stage. It is essential always to consider the patient's diagnosis, cognitive level, agitation level, contraindications & precautions.

COGNITIVE STAGE: "WHAT DO I DO?"

I. **PATIENT RELIES ON:**
- Vision and Demonstration

II. **PATIENT NEEDS:**
- Guidance and direction to pay attention to critical details of a task.

III. **FEEDBACK TYPE:**
- KR and KR-bandwidth mostly with KP intermittently and provided after every trial early f/b faded.

IV. **WHAT ENVIRONMENT TYPES:**
- Closed environments

V. **WHAT PRACTICE TIME:**
- Distributed practice

VI. **WHAT TYPE OF PRACTICE:**
- Blocked practice

VII. **WHAT PRACTICE ORDER:**
- Blocked order followed by serial and random order

VIII. **PART OR WHOLE TRAINING:**
- Part training, if possible

CHAPTER 45

ASSOCIATIVE STAGE: "HOW DO I DO THE TASK?"

I. **PATIENT RELIES ON:**
   - Proprioception and Introspection "feeling the movement."

II. **PATIENT NEEDS:**
   - Less augmented feedback and more practice

III. **FEEDBACK TYPE:**
   - Use knowledge of results (KR) and performance (KP), but limit feedback to only providing necessary feedback to improve performance/avoid faulty movement patterns.

IV. **WHAT ENVIRONMENT TYPES:**
   - Closed environments with progression to open environment

V. **WHAT PRACTICE TIME:**
   - Distributed practice as needed.

VI. **WHAT TYPE OF PRACTICE:**
   - Random practice

VII. **WHAT PRACTICE ORDER:**
   - Variable practice order, serial, and random order

VIII. **PART OR WHOLE TRAINING:**
   - Part training as needed. Focus on whole training if possible.

SECTION II

AUTONOMOUS STAGE: "HOW TO MASTER THE TASK?"

I. PATIENT RELIES ON:
- Self-evaluation, conscious awareness of performance

II. PATIENT NEEDS:
- Higher level practice with distractions

III. FEEDBACK TYPE:
- Only occasionally, KP and KR, when errors are consistent.

IV. WHAT ENVIRONMENT TYPES:
- Open environments

V. WHAT PRACTICE TIME:
- Massed Practice

VI. WHAT TYPE OF PRACTICE:
- Random practice

VII. WHAT PRACTICE ORDER:
- Random practice order

VIII. PART OR WHOLE TRAINING:
- Whole training only

CHAPTER 46

TRAUMATIC BRAIN INJURY

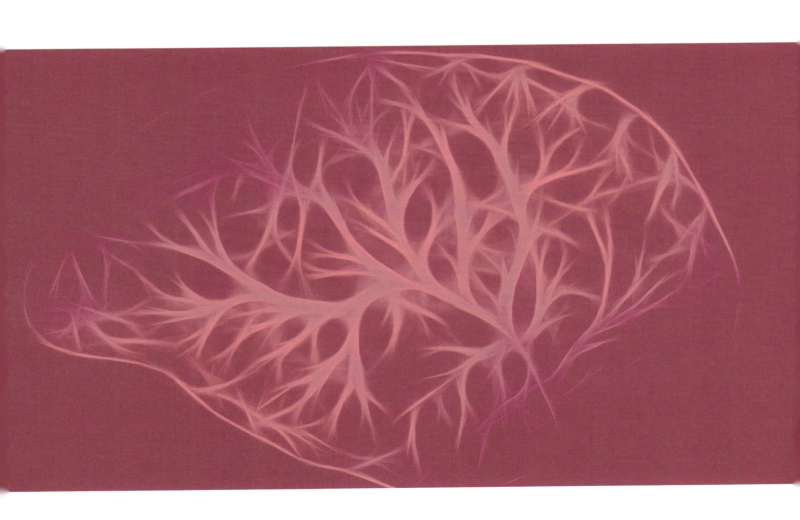

GLASGOW COMA SCALE (GCS)[15]

The GCS scale is a reliable neurological scale that objectively **assesses a person's consciousness immediately post-TBI** and upon subsequent assessments. The three components of this scale are eye movement, verbal communication, and movement/motor response.

Please do not confuse the GCS with the Ranchos Los Amigos Levels of Cognitive Functioning (LOCF) scale, which examines cognitive and behavioral recovery in individuals with TBI. The LOCF scale does not address specific cognitive deficits.

GCS SCORING

The GCS is scored from 3 to 15, with 3 being the lowest (most disabled) and 15 being the highest (least disabled) score.

Severe Brain Injury: < 9

Moderate Brain Injury: 9 - 12

Mild Brain Injury: 13 – 15

INTRACRANIAL PRESSURE (ICP)

ICP exerts pressure on the brain tissues inside the cranium. We expect patients with traumatic brain injuries to have increased intracranial pressure.

Increased ICP is mainly caused by increased swelling/blood within the cranium.

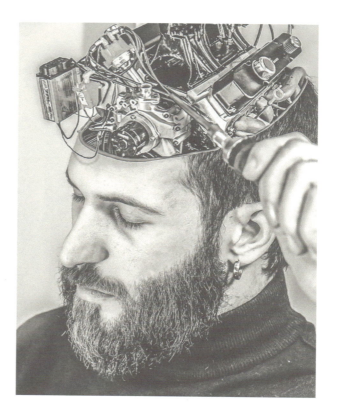

ICP MEASUREMENTS

Normal ICP: 5 - 15 mmHg

Abnormal ICP: >20 mmHg

AVOID THESE PHYSICAL THERAPY ACTIVITIES!!!

1. Cervical flexion
2. Percussion and/or Vibration
3. Coughing
4. Trendelenburg position

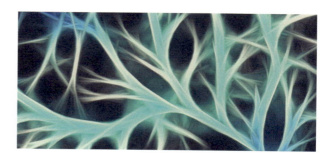

CHAPTER 46

HETEROTOPIC OSSIFICATION (HO)[16]

HO is the abnormal growth of bone in the non-skeletal tissues, including muscle, tendons, or other soft tissue. When HO develops, new bone grows three times the normal rate, resulting in jagged, painful joints.

Patients who suffer from a TBI and are immobilized for prolonged periods often develop HO. These patients can display diminished joint mobility, decreased range of motion, and increasingly painful joints.

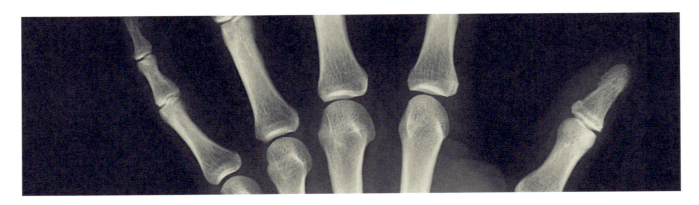

DIAGNOSTIC IMAGING METHODS

Radiographs (X-ray)
- It can take 4-6 weeks before clinicians can visualize HO with this tool.

Ultrasonography
- Detection of HO is two weeks earlier than radiograph.

Bone Scintigraphy (Bone Scan)
- Can provide information on early phases (hyperemia & blood pooling) of HO.

PHYSICAL THERAPY INTERVENTION

- Alert the physician and medical team of the suspected HO immediately when found in the acute or outpatient setting.
- Therapists can perform Pre-op PT to preserve motion around the lesion.
- ROM exercises that include:
    o PROM, AAROM, AROM, and gentle strengthening exercises are permitted but should not provoke pain.

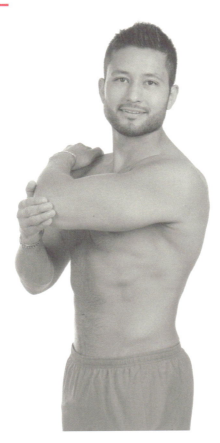

"INVENIUM VIAM AUT FACIUM"

—COACH K

CHAPTER 47

VESTIBULAR SPECIAL TESTING

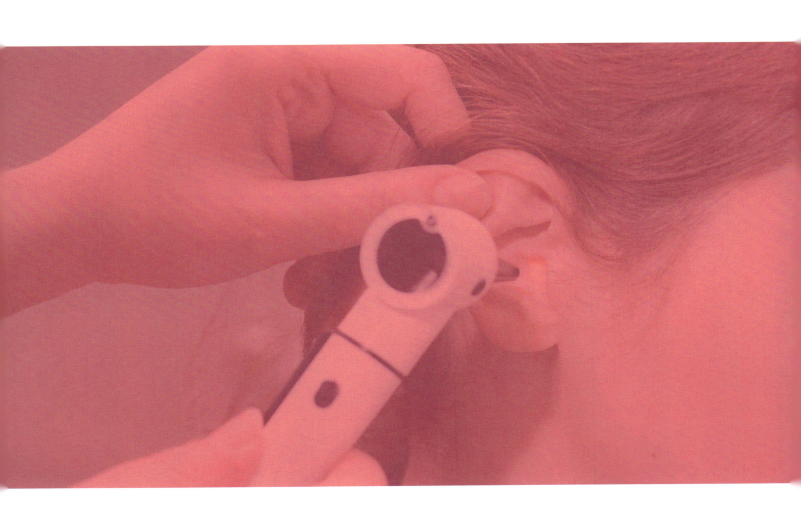

SECTION II

TYPES OF HEARING LOSS

SENSORINEURAL HEARING LOSS

This hearing loss results from a dysfunction in the inner ear, cochlea, or vestibulocochlear nerve (CN VIII).

MAJOR CAUSES	MAJOR COMPLAINTS
Ototoxicity (chronic use of antibiotics) Normal aging Traumatic Brain Injury (TBI) Exposure to loud noises/explosions Congenital dysfunction Acoustic neuroma Meniere's disease	Soft sounds are difficult to hear, and loud sounds are muffled. Most commonly, high-pitched frequency sounds are inaudible.

CONDUCTION HEARING LOSS

This hearing loss happens when something blocks the passage of sound in either the ear canal or the middle ear.

MAJOR CAUSES	MAJOR COMPLAINTS
Accumulation of ear wax Otitis media (middle ear infection) Otosclerosis (abnormal bone growth in the middle ear) Cholesteatoma (abnormal growth of tissue in the middle ear)	Soft sounds are difficult to hear regardless of the pitch level. Loud sounds may present muffled.

CHAPTER 47

TESTS FOR HEARING LOSS[17]

WEBER'S TEST

A screening test used to evaluate the presence of sensorineural and/or bone conductive hearing loss by comparing the difference in sound intensity between both ears.

Procedure

- A 256 Hz or 512 Hz tuning fork is struck and placed on top of the head equidistant from the patient's ears.
- The clinician asks the patient to report in which ear the sound is heard louder.
- Negative Test
    o The test is negative if the sound is heard equally in both ears.
- Positive Test
    o This finding is consistent with conductive hearing loss if the sound is heard louder on the affected side.
    o This finding is consistent with sensorineural hearing loss in the affected ear if the sound is heard louder on the unaffected side.

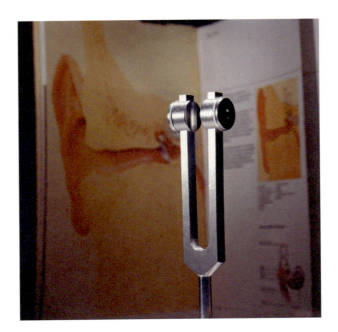

RINNE'S TEST

- Rinne's test evaluates hearing loss in one ear by comparing sounds transmitted by air conduction to those transmitted by bone conduction through the mastoid.
- Therefore, Rinne's test primarily assesses unilateral bone conductive hearing loss and should be accompanied by Weber's Test.
- The Weber's Test allows prompt detection of conductive and sensorineural hearing loss.

Procedure

- Strike a 512 Hz tuning fork and place it on the mastoid bone of the suspected side, then ask the patient to report when they can no longer hear the sound.
- When the patient can no longer hear the sound, quickly place the still-vibrating tuning fork 1-2 cm from the auditory canal.
- The therapist asks the patient to report when they can no longer hear the sound.
- Negative Test
    o The patient should be able to hear the tuning fork when held 1-2 cm outside of the ear (pinna) after they can no longer hear it when held against the mastoid.
- Positive Test
    o If the patient doesn't hear the tuning fork when moved from the mastoid to the outside of the ear, it indicates conductive hearing loss.
    o If the patient can hear the tuning fork outside the ear longer than when held against the mastoid BUT reports that the sound has stopped before the tuning fork quits vibrating, this indicates sensorineural hearing loss.

"THE NPTE IS LIKE A BOXING MATCH...SOMETIMES YOU'LL GET HIT, BUT WHAT TRULY COUNTS IS HOW MANY TIMES YOU HIT BACK."

–COACH K

CHAPTER 48

VESTIBULAR REHAB

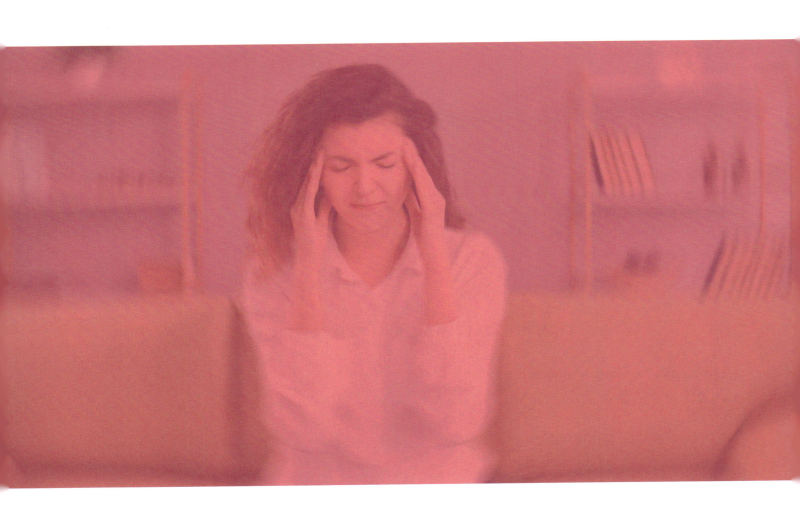

SECTION II

BENIGN PAROXYSMAL POSITIONAL VERTIGO

BPPV, a peripheral vestibular condition, causes the sensation of vertigo (room spinning), nystagmus, and nausea/vomiting when positioning the head in specific ways or postures.

CANALITHIASIS INTERVENTIONS

Epley's Maneuver

The therapist moves the patient's head into different positions in a sequence that will move the debris (otoconia) out of the involved semi-circular canals and into the vestibule.

1. The head is rotated towards the affected ear.
2. The patient's head is rotated 45 degrees to each side and 30 degrees of cervical extension when supine.
3. This intervention is repeated 3-5 times, up to 3 times per day.
4. This continues until the symptoms are resolved for two consecutive days.

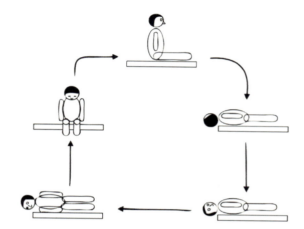

Brandt-Daroff

1. The patient's head is rotated to 45 degrees while sitting at the edge of the bed.
2. The patient quickly lies down to the side opposite of the rotation.
3. The position is held for 1 minute.
4. The patient then sits back up at the edge of the bed, rotates the head in the opposite direction to 45 degrees, and quickly lies down to the side opposite the rotation.
5. This is repeated 5-10 times, 3x a day.

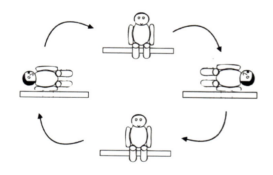

CUPULOLITHIASIS INTERVENTIONS

Liberatory Semont Maneuver

1. The patient's head is rotated to 45 degrees while sitting at the edge of the bed. The patient quickly lies down to the side opposite of the rotation x 1 minute.
2. Then, the patient is quickly moved to lying down on the opposite shoulder with the head kept in the same position throughout.
3. This is repeated 5-10 times, 2-3x per day.

UNILATERAL VESTIBULAR HYPOFUNCTION (UVH)[18]

- UVH is a pathology affecting one side of the vestibular system that causes a loss of signaling or diminished signaling to the brain.
- This condition is characterized by nausea/vomiting, nystagmus, vertigo, disequilibrium, and postural instability.

VESTIBULAR REHABILITATION

Habituation Exercises

- Habituation training aims to reduce the patient's symptoms through neural adaptation.
- This occurs by repeatedly provoking the undesired response.
- The therapist finds the provoking positions that induce mild or moderate dizziness.
- The patient is instructed to move into and out of those positions for 3-5 repetitions, 2-3x per day.

Example Interventions

- Go from flat on your back to your left side.
- Go from your left side to your right side.
- From a sitting position, touch the nose to the left knee.
- From a sitting position, touch the nose to the right knee.
- From a sitting position, move your head up and down.
- Sitting on the side of the bed, turn your head to the right and lie down quickly.
- Sitting on the side of the bed, turn your head to the left and lie down quickly.

GAZE STABILITY TRAINING (VOR)	
VOR x1	VOR x2
Move the head horizontally or vertically while maintaining focus on an object.	Move the head and target in opposing directions while maintaining gaze on the target and target in focus.

BILATERAL VESTIBULAR HYPOFUNCTION (BVH)

- BVH is a pathology affecting both sides of the vestibular system that causes a loss of signaling or diminished signaling to the brain.
- This condition is characterized as having disequilibrium and gait ataxia.
- Vertigo and nystagmus **ARE NOT** expected with this condition.
- Therefore, interventions focusing on decreasing vertigo, such as habituation, are not indicated.

VESTIBULAR REHABILITATION

GAZE STABILITY TRAINING (VOR)	
VOR x1	VOR x2
Move the head horizontally or vertically while maintaining focus on an object.	Move the head and target in opposing directions while maintaining gaze on the target and target in focus.

Goal of Gaze Stabilization Training

- To improve the patient's ability to maintain a target in focus and disallow blurring of the target.
- The patient should start with VORx1 first and then progress to VORx2.
- To increase the challenge, the clinician can modify the background by changing the background color, texture, or pattern.

Postural Stability Training

- Postural stability training involves utilizing intact balance systems such as vision and somatosensation to compensate for the impaired vestibular system.
- Common interventions include standing on foam with eyes open, standing on level ground with eyes closed, tandem stance, and standing with a narrow base of support.

SECTION II REFERENCES

1. O'Sullivan, Susan B., Schmitz, Thomas J.Fulk, George D. (©2014) Physical rehabilitation /Philadelphia: F.A. Davis Co
2. O'Sullivan, Susan B., Schmitz, Thomas J.Fulk, George D. (©2014) Physical rehabilitation /Philadelphia: F.A. Davis Co.,
3. O'Sullivan, Susan B., Schmitz, Thomas J. Fulk, George D. Physical Rehabilitation. Philadelphia: F.A. Davis Co., 2014.
4. O'Sullivan, S. B., & Schmitz, T. J. (2007). Physical rehabilitation. Philadelphia, PA: F.A. Davis. Pg 116-117, 179
5. Martin, S., & Kessler, M. (2016). Neurologic interventions for physical therapy. St. Louis, MO: Elsevier Saunders.
6. http://www.strokecenter.org/professionals/stroke-diagnosis/stroke-syndromes/lateral-medullary-syndrome-wallenberg- syndrome/ National Institute of Neurological Disorders and Stroke: Wallenberg Syndrome. https://www.ninds.nih.gov/disorders/all- disorders/wallenbergs-syndrome-information-page(accessed 4 May 2017).
7. Goodman, C. C., & Fuller, K. S. (2009). Pathology: Implications for the physical therapist. St. Louis, Mo: Saunders/Elsevier. Reference: Goodman, C. C., & Snyder, T. E. K. (2007). Differential diagnosis for physical therapists: Screening for referral. St. Louis, Mo: Saunders/Elsevier
8. Magee, D. J. (2008). Orthopedic physical assessment. St. Louis, Mo: Saunders Elsevier.
9. Martin, S., & Kessler, M. (2016). Neurologic interventions for physical therapy. St. Louis, MO: Elsevier Saunders.Umphred, D. A. (2013). Umphred's Neurological Rehabilitation. St. Louis, Mo: Elsevier/Mosby.
10. Martin, S., & Kessler, M. (2016). Neurologic interventions for physical therapy. St. Louis, MO: Elsevier Saunders. Umphred, D. A. (2013). Umphred's Neurological Rehabilitation. St. Louis, Mo: Elsevier/Mosby.
11. Martin, Suzanne., Kessler, Mary. Neurologic Interventions For Physical Therapy. 2016. 3rd Edition, pp 257 -262
12. Sullivan, S.B. Physical Rehabilitation. 6th edition. Pgs 674, 695
13. https://spinabifidaassociation.org/wp-content/uploads/2015/07/HOW-SB-LESIONS-IMPACT-DAILY-FUNCTION1.pdf
14. O'Sullivan, S.B. Physical Rehabilitation. 6th edition pgs 396-401, 407-414
15. O'Sullivan, S. B., & Schmitz, T. J. (2007). Physical rehabilitation. Philadelphia, PA: F .A. Davis.
16. (1) Mavrogenis AF, Soucacos PN, Papagelopoulos PJ. Heterotopic Ossification Revisited. Orthopedics. 2011Jan;34(3):177.
    (2) Firoozabadi R, Alton T, Sagi HC. Heterotopic Ossification in Acetabular Fracture Surgery. Journal of the American Academy of Orthopaedic Surgeons. 2017;25(2):117–24.
    (3) Bossche LV, Vanderstraeten G. Heterotopic ossification: a review. J Rehabil Med 2005; 37: 129-136.5. Pape HC et al. Current concepts in the development of heterotopic ossification. Journ Bone and Joint Surg 2004; 86: 783-787.
17. O'Sullivan, S. B., & Schmitz, T. J. (2007). Physical rehabilitation. Philadelphia, PA: F.A. Davis Magee, David J. Orthopedic Physical Assessment. St. Louis, Mo: Saunders Elsevier, 2008.
18. O'Sullivan, S.B. Physical Rehabilitation. 6th Edition. Pgs. 980-90

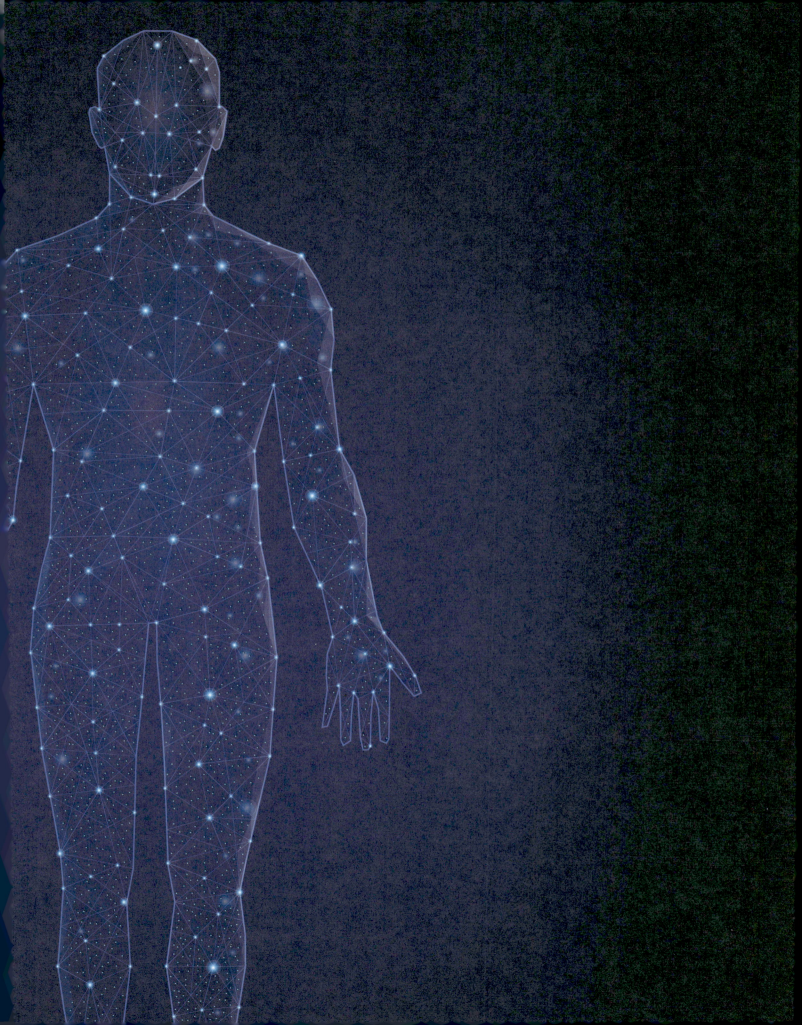

SECTION III

CARDIOPULMONARY CHEAT SHEETS

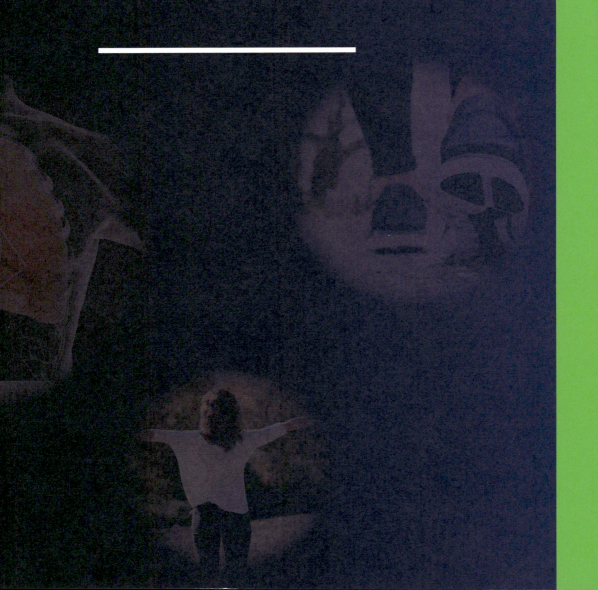

CHAPTER 49

6-MINUTE WALK TEST

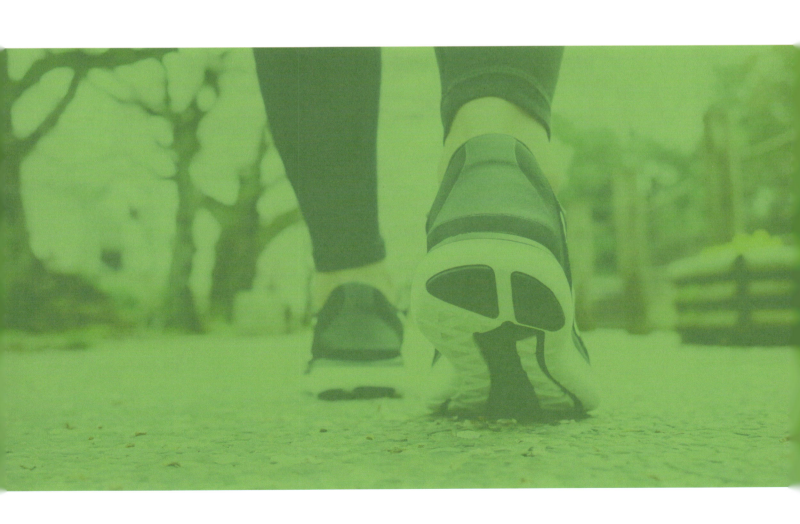

6-MINUTE WALK TEST (6MWT)[1]

WHAT IS THE 6MWT & WHAT IS THE TEST USED FOR?

The 6MWT is a valid and reliable submaximal exercise test to assess walking endurance (functional endurance) and aerobic capacity.

WHO DO I USE THIS TEST FOR? (NOT LIMITED TO:)

1. Pretreatment and post-treatment comparisons
2. Lung transplantation
3. Lung surgery
4. Pulmonary rehabilitation
5. COPD
6. Pulmonary hypertension
7. Congestive Heart Failure (CHF)
8. Cystic fibrosis
9. Peripheral vascular disease
10. Fibromyalgia
11. Older patients
12. Predictor of morbidity and mortality

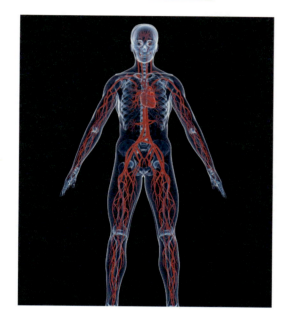

WHAT IS THE TESTING PROCEDURE?

- The testing environment consists of a hallway or open area 100 feet long. A chair is placed at each end of the walkway, and floor markers are placed every 3 meters.
- The patient is instructed to walk as far as possible for 6 minutes. The patient can slow down, stop, and rest as necessary.
- The patient may lean against the wall while resting but resume walking as soon as they are able.
- The distance the patient traveled in the 6 minutes allotted is recorded.

CHAPTER 49

WHAT ARE SOME NPTE CURVEBALLS RELATED TO THIS OUTCOME MEASURE?

- The patient is allowed to use an assistive device. However, the device should be the least restrictive without jeopardizing the patient's safety.
- The patient is alerted after each minute how much time remains. For example, "You have 5 minutes left".
- Non-standardized encouragement is prohibited.
- Acceptable verbal encouragement includes, "Keep up the good work" or "You are doing well."
- The therapist should walk a half step behind the patient rather than beside or in front to avoid setting the patient's pace.

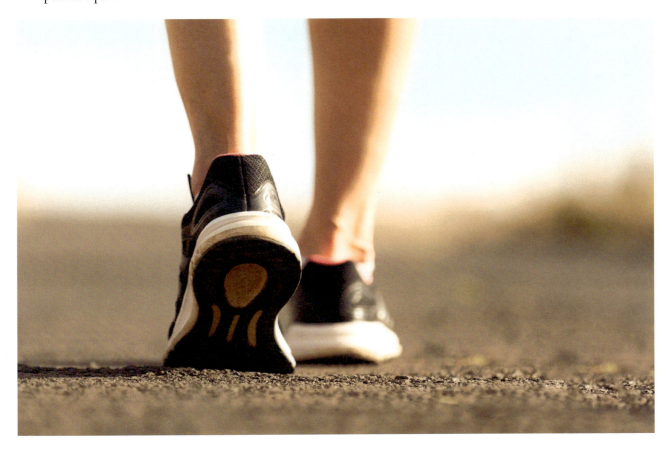

WHY CHOOSE SIX-MINUTE WALK TEST OVER VO2MAX?

- No expensive equipment is required.
- Can perform 6MWT with patients who are ill, elderly, or post-surgical.
- Results of the 6MWT are highly correlated with functional activity.

"SUCCESS LEAVES CLUES. IF WE REPLICATE WHAT'S SUCCESSFUL, WE CAN START TO GET AMAZING IMPROVEMENTS IN WHAT WE DESIRE."

– COACH K

CHAPTER 50

ALTITUDE & CARDIOPULMONARY

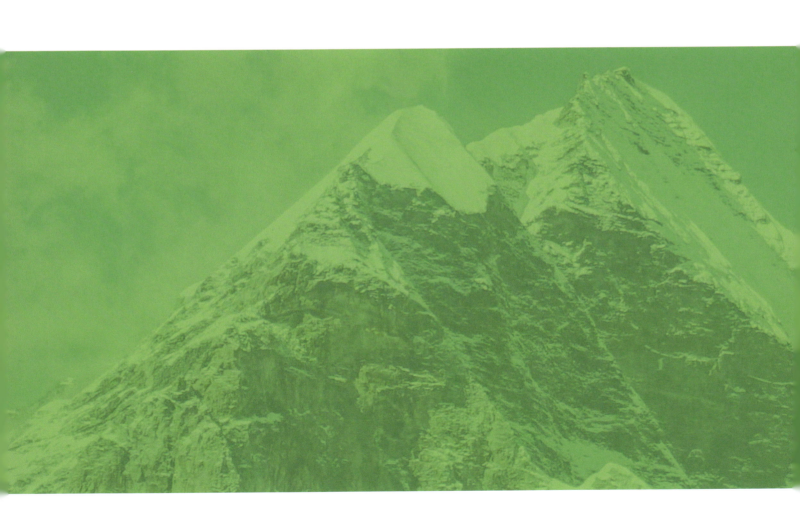

SECTION III

RESPONSE TO HIGH-ALTITUDE[2]

Changes in altitude are known to have a significant impact on the cardiopulmonary system and physiology.

High altitude is 1,500–3,500 meters (4,900–11,500 ft).

> "At high altitudes, atmospheric pressure is low, and the partial pressure of oxygen (PaO2) is low."

ACUTE REACTION TO HIGH ALTITUDE

INCREASED HEART RATE	DECREASED EXERCISE PERFORMANCE
INCREASED CARDIAC OUTPUT	DECREASED STROKE VOLUME
INCREASED BLOOD PRESSURE	DECREASED ARTERIAL PaCO2
INCREASED VENTILATION	

*Stroke volume can remain relatively unchanged depending on the significance of the altitude change.

ALTITUDE SICKNESS

Altitude sickness is a cluster of signs and symptoms caused by rapid exposure to low amounts of oxygen at high altitudes.

COMMON SIGNS & SYMPTOMS TO KNOW

Headache, lethargy, nausea/vomiting, dyspnea, peripheral edema, epistaxis, dizziness, insomnia

"I DON'T NEED YOU TO BE PERFECT. I JUST NEED YOU TO GIVE YOUR B.E.S.T... BETTER EVERY SINGLE TIME."

— COACH K

CHAPTER 51

AQUATIC THERAPY

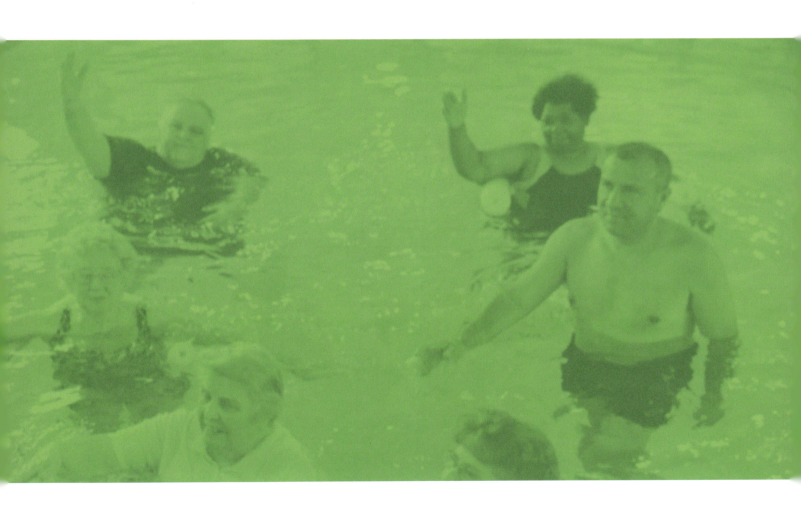

SECTION III

AQUATIC THERAPY

THE RESPIRATORY SYSTEM

Hydrostatic pressure is the force applied by water against the walls of a submerged object. When the body is submerged above the Xiphoid process, hydrostatic pressure increases the difficulty of breathing, which can cause an increased respiratory rate.

NPTE Note: Patients with dyspnea should avoid submersion above the Xiphoid process.

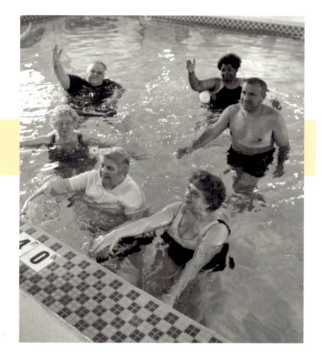

THE NEUROLOGIC SYSTEM

Water temperature is the leading factor that impacts neurologic functioning in the aquatic environment. Warm water tends to be relaxing and can have superior effects on hypertonia and spasticity. However, cool/cold water tends to be stimulating and invigorating.

NPTE Note: Conditions such as Multiple Sclerosis, considered demyelinating pathologies, should avoid water temperatures above 84 degrees Fahrenheit.

THE MUSCULOSKELETAL SYSTEM

Water temperature is one of the most significant factors that impact muscle function. Warm water increases vasodilation to exercising muscles and reduces fatiguability. Strength gains have been reported with resistance exercises underwater using the principle of hydrostatic drag. Drag is the water's resistance to a body or object in motion.

CHAPTER 51

THE CARDIOVASCULAR SYSTEM

The CV system is greatly impacted by water immersion. If the water temperature is above 95.9 degrees F (warm), peripheral vasodilation will occur. If the water temperature is below 80.6 degrees F (cold), peripheral vasoconstriction will occur.

WHAT HAPPENS TO THE HEART RATE?[3]

Immersion in warm to hot water will increase the heart rate. Water that is set to body temperature has a neutral effect on the heart rate.

Immersion in cold water stimulates a physiological response called the diving reflex. The patient will exhibit a decreased heart rate, peripheral vasoconstriction, and cardiac output. This response occurs to reduce O2 demand and preserve the vital organs.

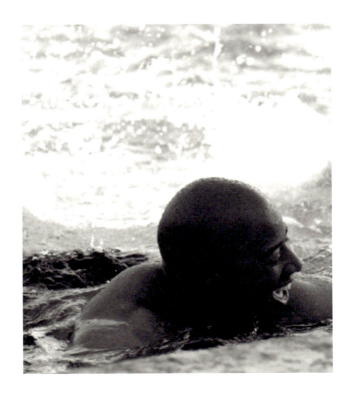

WHAT HAPPENS TO THE BLOOD PRESSURE?

Immersion in cool water temperatures stimulates the diving reflex, which increases peripheral vasoconstriction. Since blood pressure is heavily dependent on blood vessel diameter, the blood pressure increases as the blood vessels constrict. During immersion in warm to hot waters, the blood pressure decreases secondary to rapid peripheral vasodilation.

CHAPTER 52

ARTERIAL INSUFFICIENCY

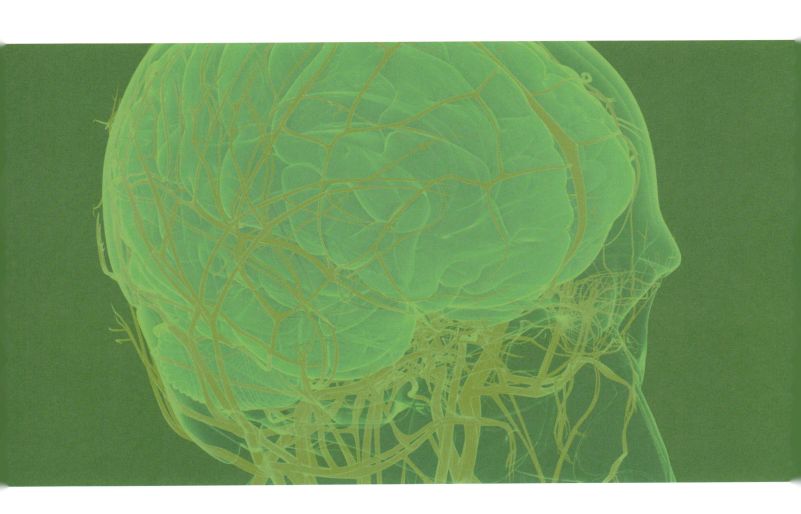

SECTION III

ARTERIAL INSUFFICIENCY[4]

Arterial insufficiency refers to a lack of adequate blood flow to a region or regions of the body.

QUICK FACTS

Arterial insufficiency is common in patients with diabetes mellitus, hypertension, obesity, and smoking. Most experts agree that the most effective intervention is smoking cessation education followed by exercise and weight control.

Arteriosclerosis Obliterans is a peripheral manifestation of atherosclerosis characterized by intermittent claudication, rest pain, and trophic changes.

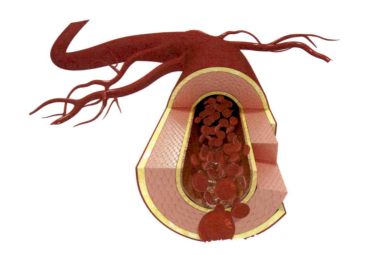

ANKLE-BRACHIAL INDEX VALUES	
ABI RANGE	CLINICAL INTERPRETATION
>1.2	Falsely Elevated, Arterial Disease, Diabetes
1.19 – 0.95	Normal
0.94 – 0.75	Mild Arterial Disease + Intermittent Claudication
0.74 – 0.50	Moderate Arterial Disease, Rest pain
<0.50	Severe Arterial Disease

SIGNS & SYMPTOMS MNEMONIC

Pale (pallor)

Abnormal nail growth

Little leg or foot hair

Lateral malleolar wounds

Overly dry and shiny skin

Rest pain or intermittent claudication

"THE PAIN OF DISCIPLINE IS LESS THAN THE PAIN OF REGRET."

— COACH K

CHAPTER 53

BLOOD GASES

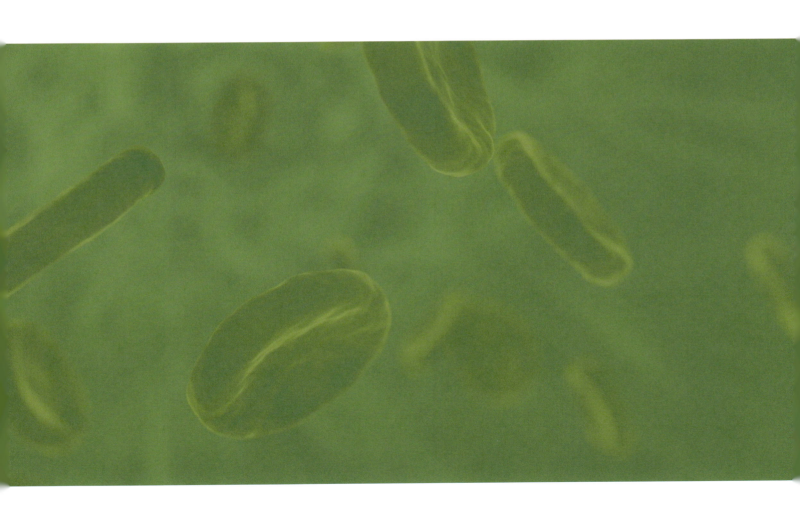

BLOOD GASES

RESPIRATORY ACIDOSIS

"CARBS"

Confusion
Agitation
Restlessness
Blurred vision
Seizures

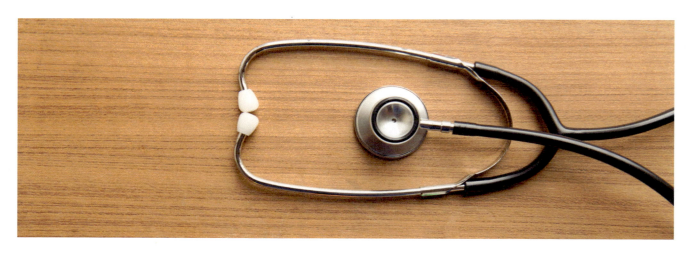

RESPIRATORY ALKALOSIS

"NO CARDS"

Numbness/Tingling
Orthostatic Hypotension
Confusion
Anxiety
Rapid breathing
Dizziness
Seizures

METABOLIC ACIDOSIS

"SHAMED"

S tupor
H yperkalemia
A rrhythmias
M uscle twitching
E mesis
D ecreased cardiac output

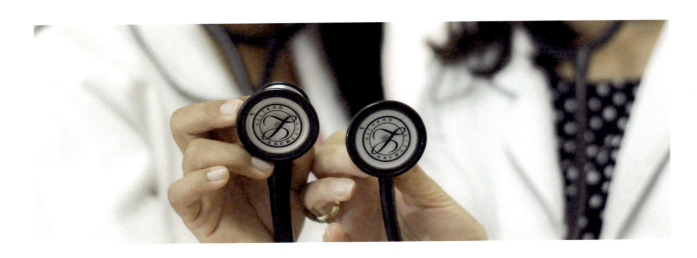

METABOLIC ALKALOSIS

The Quad T's

T etany
T achycardia
T remors
T ingling

"IT IS DURING OUR DARKEST MOMENTS THAT WE MUST FOCUS ON THE LIGHT"

— COACH K

CHAPTER 54

EKG INTERPRETATION

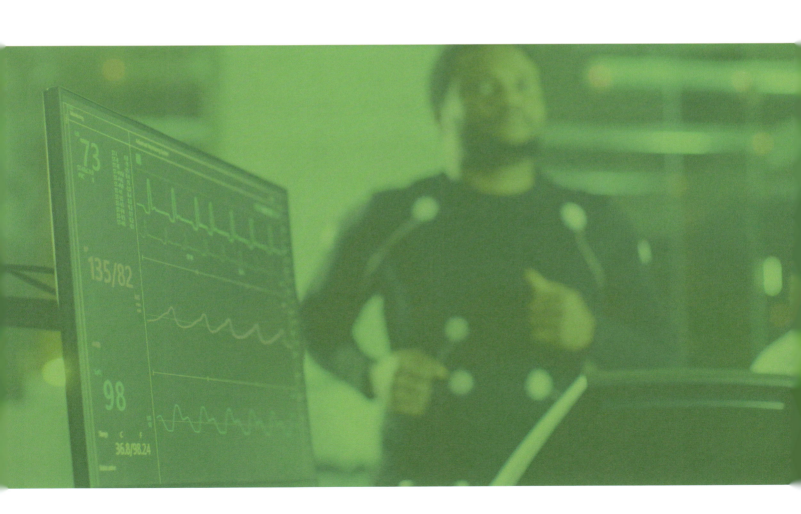

SECTION III

EKG/ECG INTERPRETATION

TOP EKG ABNORMAL READINGS

FIRST DEGREE AV NODE BLOCK

A potentially impaired AV node causes a delayed contraction of the ventricles. First-degree AV node blocks can be normal in athletes.

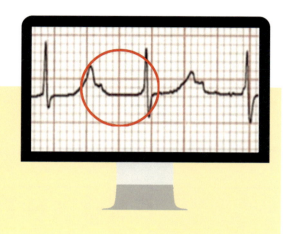

CLINICAL NOTES:
1. The P-wave is buried inside the T-wave with a delayed QRS complex that follows.
2. Can be normal in some populations and is benign when the abnormality does not create symptoms.
3. Exercise the patient as normal but monitor vitals closely, especially with changes in exercise intensity.

SECOND DEGREE AV NODE BLOCK (TYPE 1)

This abnormality can also be called the Mobitz I or Wenckebach AV node block. This block is characterized by progressively longer delays between the P-wave and the QRS complex until the point of a missed QRS complex (i.e., ventricular contraction).

CLINICAL NOTES:
1. Can be classified as a physiological anomaly in many cases and is considered benign.
2. No further medical treatment is necessary if the patient is asymptomatic.
3. If the patient is symptomatic, immediately send them to the physician.
4. These patients may require a pacemaker.

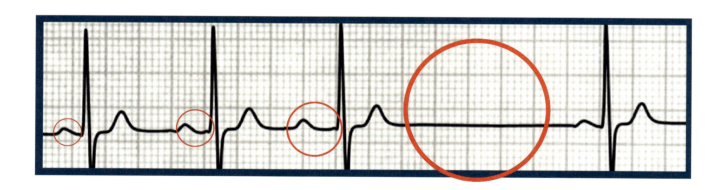

CHAPTER 54

SECOND DEGREE AV NODE BLOCK (TYPE 2)

This abnormality can also be called the Mobitz II AV node block. This block is characterized by intermittent skipping of QRS complexes.

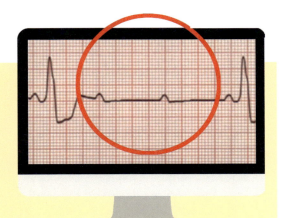

CLINICAL NOTES:
1. All patients will undergo a pacemaker or heart procedure.
2. If this abnormality is found without a pacemaker and with symptoms present, call EMS
3. If this abnormality is found without symptoms, stop exercise and refer to a physician immediately.
4. A Mobitz Type II can quickly become a third-degree AV node block without proper medical treatment.

THIRD DEGREE AV NODE BLOCK[5]

This severe EKG abnormality occurs when there is no longer a relationship between the P-wave and QRS complex. The heart is no longer beating in synchrony, which causes a rapid decline in cardiac output.

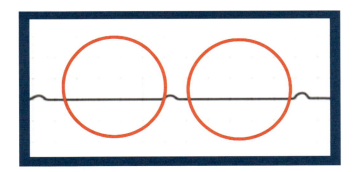

CLINICAL NOTES:
1. Call EMS if found in the clinic.
2. This EKG abnormality rapidly changes to asystole, which means without contraction.[5]

ST-SEGMENT ELEVATION

An increase in the ST-segment relative to the isoelectric line. In many cases, an ST-segment elevation indicates myocardial infarction, also known as a STEMI.

CLINICAL NOTES:
1. Greater than 1mm ST-segment elevation is significant and indicates myocardial infarction.
2. If a true STEMI is observed, the exercise should be terminated, and EMS alerted.
3. Sometimes, EKG leads can detach or move while exercising. Ensure proper lead connection if a STEMI is observed on the monitor without other symptoms.

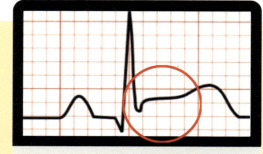

ST-SEGMENT DEPRESSION

A decrease in the ST-segment relative to the isoelectric line. There are many causes of this depression. However, the most common cause is myocardial ischemia or lack of blood flow to a heart region.

CLINICAL NOTES:
1. When exercising a patient, > 2mm ST segment depression is considered significant. Stop the exercise and monitor the vitals. (Warning: This recommendation is for exercise, not the exercise tolerance test.)
2. When exercising a patient with 0-2mm ST segment depression, monitor vitals and use clinical judgment on whether to stop or continue exercise (i.e., additional signs/symptoms).

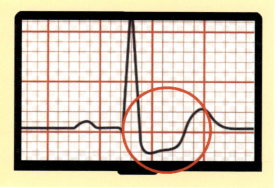

CHAPTER 54

ATRIAL FIBRILLATION

Irregularly irregular heartbeat characterized by a highly frequent and erratic quivering of the atria.

CLINICAL NOTES:
1. Monitoring is recommended for all cardiac patients.
2. New onset of A-Fib should be reported immediately to the physician.
3. Patients with A-Fib should take blood thinners to reduce the risk of stroke.
4. Atrial fibrillation is not a medical emergency unless life-threatening signs/symptoms arise (i.e., loss of consciousness, confusion).

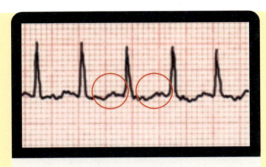

PRE-VENTRICULAR CONTRACTION (PVC)

Bizarre-looking QRS complexes without a preceding P-wave. It can be normal if isolated and infrequent.

Common Types:
Couplet PVCs: Two Consecutive PVCs
Triplet PVCs: Three Consecutive PVCs
Bigeminy: Every other QRS complex is a PVC
Trigeminy: Every third QRS complex is a PVC

CLINICAL NOTES:
1. If one PVC is isolated, continue exercising and monitor vitals.
2. Call the emergency medical services if six (6) PVCs are found in one strip.
3. hree (3) consecutive PVCs in a row is known as V-tach and requires an EMS call
4. A PVC that lands directly on a T-wave impairs the heart's ability to fill up with blood. If this is found on the EKG, the therapist should call EMS.

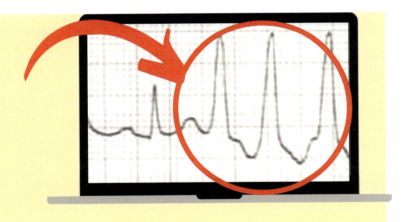

283

"THIS IS JUST ANOTHER CHAPTER IN YOUR LIFE, NOT THE END OF YOUR STORY."

— COACH K

CHAPTER 55

EXERCISE RESPONSES

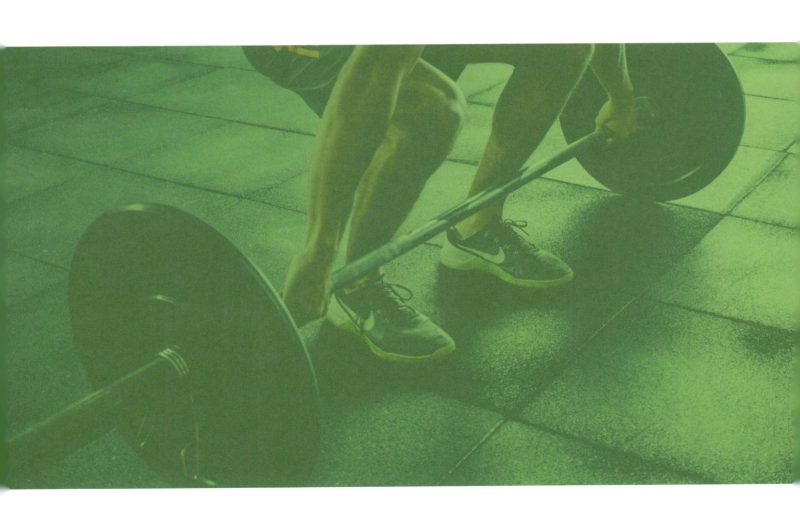

EXERCISE RESPONSES

BLOOD PRESSURE

Blood pressure (BP) is the pressure of circulating blood on arterial walls and is categorized as systolic and diastolic blood pressure on the NPTE.

Systolic Blood Pressure (SBP) is the pressure on the arterial walls during ventricular contraction.

Diastolic Blood Pressure (DBP) is the pressure on the arterial walls during ventricular relaxation.

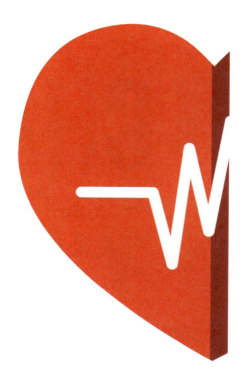

NORMAL RESPONSE TO EXERCISE

- Heart and respiratory rates increase with increasing workload.
- SBP increases by 10 mmHg per MET of increasing workload.
- DBP remains relatively constant but can change to +/- 10 mmHg from resting pressure.
- Upper extremity exercise is 30-40% less O2 demand than lower extremity exercise unless compared to the same workload.

HYPOTENSIVE RESPONSE

A hypotensive response to exercise can signify myocardial ischemia or left ventricular dysfunction.
A decrease in SBP >10mmHg
AND/OR
A decrease in DBP >10mmHg with increasing workload

BLUNTED RESPONSE

A blunted response to exercise is a failure of your SBP to rise or a rise of less than <8 mmHg per MET of increasing workload.

A blunted response is typically due to using beta-blockers or anti-hypertensive medications, which cause vasodilation, reduced cardiac contractility, and/or blunted heart rate and blood pressure response.

HYPERTENSIVE RESPONSE TO EXERCISE

- A DBP of greater than 110 mmHg
- An Increase in DBP > 10 mmHg during exercise
- A SBP of greater than 260 mmHg

BLOOD PRESSURE GUIDELINES[6]

BLOOD PRESSURE CATEGORY	SYSTOLIC (mmHg)		DIASTOLIC (mmHg)
NORMAL	<120	and	<80
ELEVATED	120 – 129	and	<80
HYPERTENSION STAGE I	130 – 139	or	80 – 89
HYPERTENSION STAGE II	≥140	or	≥90
HYPERTENSIVE CRISIS *Consult your MD immediately*	>180	and/or	>120

"STOP DWELLING ON THE PROBLEM & START CREATING THE SOLUTION"

–COACH K

CHAPTER 56

HEART SOUNDS

HEART SOUNDS

THE TOP NPTE HEART SOUNDS

S1 "THE LUB"

This sound is best heard over the apex of the heart using the bell or diaphragm of the stethoscope. This sound is heard during systole.

The S1 heart sound is low-pitched and is heard because of the turbulence created when the tricuspid and mitral valves close (systole)

S2 "THE DUB"

This sound is best heard over the base of the heart and at the beginning of the diastole.

The S2 heart sound is produced by the closure of the aortic and pulmonic semilunar valves immediately before diastole.

S3 VENTRICULAR GALLOP

This sound is best heard over the apex of the heart using the bell of the stethoscope.

The S3 heart sound occurs just after the S2 heart sound as the mitral valve opens, leading to passive filling of the left ventricle.

The S3 sound is caused by a large amount of blood striking a weakened, distended, or lean heart tissue.

S3 is normal in well-trained athletes, children, and pregnant females. This sound can be pathological and can indicate systolic congestive heart failure.

S4 ATRIAL GALLOP

This sound is best heard over the apex of the heart.

The S4 heart sound occurs just before the S1 sounds when the atria contract to force blood into the left ventricle.

The S4 sound is caused by a large amount of blood striking a non-compliant/stiff or thickened left ventricle.

S4 is almost always abnormal and is an essential sign of diastolic heart failure, myocardial infarction, or prolonged hypertension.

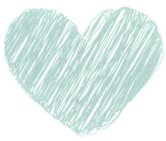

PERICARDIAL FRICTION RUB

This sound is best heard over the left sternal border using the stethoscope's diaphragm.

The rub of the pericardium lining produces the PFR sound. The pericardium is the outer layer of the heart composed of an outer fibrous layer and a double inner serous layer.

PFR is exclusively caused by pericarditis for the NPTE and has a scratchy, leather-like sound.

MITRAL STENOSIS

This sound is a low-pitched rumbling, best heard at the apex of the heart with the bell of the stethoscope. This sound is often heard after S2 through mid-diastole.

Mitral stenosis heart sounds are produced by turbulent blood flow as the blood passes from the left atrium into the left ventricle.

The most common cause of mitral valve stenosis is rheumatic fever.

AORTIC STENOSIS

This sound is best heard over the 2nd intercostal space on the right throughout the systole.

Aortic stenosis heart sounds are produced by blood passing through a narrowed diamond-shaped orifice formed from a calcified or sclerotic aortic valve.

Aortic stenosis can occur from advanced aging, wear, and tear on the aortic valve, or conditions such as rheumatic fever.

MNEUMONIC & AUSCULTATION SITES

"All People Enjoy Time Magazine"

ALL – Aorta/Aortic Valve
- 2nd intercostal space (ICS) on the right sternal border

PEOPLE – Pulmonic Semilunar Valve
- 2nd intercostal space (ICS) on the left sternal border

ENJOY – Erb's Point
- 3rd intercostal space (ICS) on the left sternal border

TIME – Tricuspid Valve
- 4th intercostal space (ICS) on the left sternal border

MAGAZINE – Mitral/Bicuspid Valve
- 5th intercostal space (ICS), mid-clavicular line on left

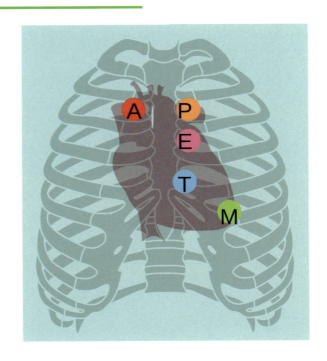

"LIFE ISN'T ABOUT WHO GETS THERE THE FASTEST… ITS ABOUT WHO ENDURES THE LONGEST."

COACH K.

CHAPTER 57

HEMODIALYSIS

WHAT IS HEMODIALYSIS?[7]

Hemodialysis occurs when a patient's blood is filtered using a specially designed blood filtration machine and dialyzer. This procedure occurs with the patient present, where the blood is removed from the patient's body, filtered, and replaced.

WHAT IS THE NPTE CONDITION TREATED WITH HEMODIALYSIS?

Chronic Renal Disease or End Stage Renal Disease (ESRD)

> **Dr. Rice's Clinical Note:** The kidneys are responsible for filtering the blood and removing chemicals and toxins, including but not limited to excess electrolytes, urea, hydrogen ions, and even excessive water. Without this proper filtration system, your patient can have fatal hypercalcemia or hyperkalemia, diabetic ketoacidosis, and metabolic acidosis, amongst many other conditions.

5 KEY NPTE FACTS ABOUT HEMODIALYSIS

1. Exercise is best performed on non-dialysis days.

2. Rate of Perceived Exertion (RPE) is the most common exercise intensity measure. The patient should stay between the 9 – 13 intensity range.

3. Weight and/or pressure should never be placed onto the arm that contains the arteriovenous fistula.

4. Blood pressure should never be taken in the arm with the arteriovenous fistula.

5. Lower extremity-based exercises can be performed during the first half of dialysis but, in most cases, should be avoided during the later parts of treatment. Exercise SHOULD NOT be performed immediately post hemodialysis.

INCREDIBLE OFFER OPPORTUNITY

Are you ready to ace the NPTE and kickstart your career as a Physical Therapist? Join over 20,000 Physical Therapy graduates who have trusted Coach K's NPTE review courses and coaching programs to guide them to success.

Under Coach K's expert guidance, you'll discover the proven formula for answering every type of NPTE question with confidence. No need to spend endless hours studying—Coach K's program is designed to make your prep efficient and effective.

Don't miss out! Limited spots are available, so act fast and scan the QR code below for more information and secure your spot in this all-inclusive program.

Your dream PT career is just one step away!

CHAPTER 58

LAB VALUES

SECTION III

EXERCISE GUIDELINES & LAB VALUES

LAB VALUE	NORMAL RANGE	EXERCISE GUIDELINES
GLUCOSE	Ideal Exercise Range: 100 – 250 mg/dl	<70 mg/dl: No exercise; give 15g carbohydrate snack. 70 – 100 mg/dl with symptoms: No exercise, give 15g carbohydrate snack, retest in 15 minutes. 70 – 100 mg/dl w/o symptoms: Exercise w/ caution, give 15g carbohydrate snack, retest in 15 minutes. 250 – 300 mg/dl w/ presence of ketones: No exercise, call EMS. 250 – 300 mg/dl w/o ketones present: Exercise cautiously; retest in 15 minutes. >300 mg/dl: No exercise permitted. Call EMS if symptoms and/or ketones are present.
HEMOGLOBIN (Hgb)	Female: 12 – 16 g/dL Male: 14 – 17 g/dL	<8 g/dL: No exercise (document & discuss with physician) 8 – 10 g/dL: Light exercise permitted; avoid aerobic exercise. 10 – 12 g/dL: Low intensity/impact exercise permitted; resistance training is permitted.
HEMATOCRIT (Hct)	Male: 42 – 52% Female: 37 – 47%	<25%: No exercise >25%: Light exercise; avoid resistive exercise permitted. >/= 30%: progression to resistive exercises
INTERNATIONAL NORMALIZED RATIO (INR)	0.9 – 1.1	>2.5: Use extreme caution and guard against falls. >3.0: Risk for hemarthrosis >4.0: Progression of exercise contraindicated; discuss with a physician

PLATELETS	150,000 – 450,000	<10,000: Transfusion: No PT Services
		<20,000: Basic ADLs, AAROM/AROM, no antigravity or resistance training permitted.
		20,000 - 30,000: Light exercises
		30,000 – 50,000: AROM, sub-max isometrics permitted, avoid prolonged stretching and resistance
		50,000 – 150,000: Minimal to moderate resistive exercises permitted
WHITE BLOOD CELLS (WBC)	$5.0 – 10.0 \ 10^9/L$	$<5.0 \times 10^9$ with fever: No exercise
		$>5.0 \times 10^9$: Light exercise permitted with progression to resistive exercise

CHAPTER 59

NPTE BIOMARKERS

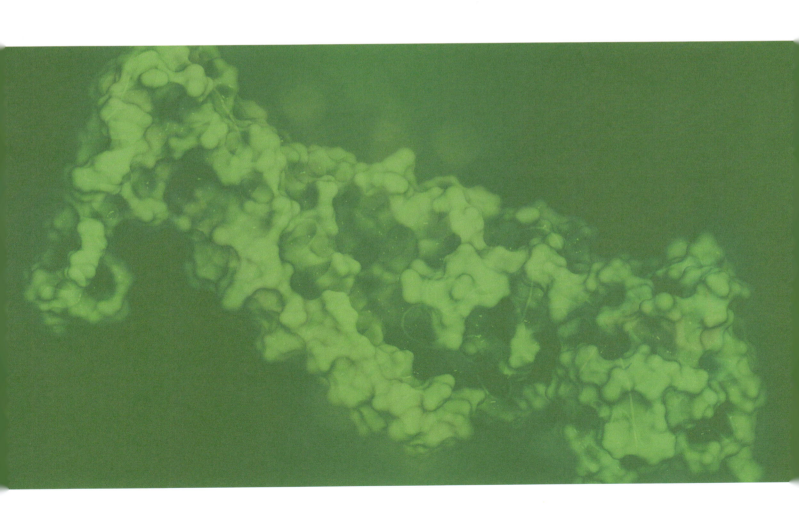

BIOMARKERS[8]

CARDIAC BIOMARKERS

CARDIAC TROPONIN

This protein is one of the most used assessed biomarkers. Troponin enters your bloodstream post-myocardial infarction (MI).

NORMAL RANGES	POST-MI LEVELS
0.0 – 0.03 ng/mL	> 0.10 ng/mL

BRAIN NATRIURETIC PEPTIDE (BNP)

BNP is a peptide hormone released during volume expansion and stress on the heart's walls. An increase in this biomarker is seen with heart failure (HF).

NORMAL RANGES	POST-MI LEVELS
< 100 pg/mL	> 100 – 300 pg/mL Class I HF
	> 300 pg/mL Class II HF
	> 600 pg/mL Class III HF
	> 900 pg/mL Class IV HF

INFLAMMATORY BIOMARKERS

C-REACTIVE PROTEIN (CRP)

This protein biomarker is made by the liver and is produced in excess when an inflammatory process occurs in the body. Conditions such as arthritis, rheumatic disorders, Lupus, vasculitis, meningitis, or other visceral inflammatory diseases cause elevated CRP.

NORMAL RANGES	ELEVATED
<3.0 mg/L	>3.0 mg/L

Special Note: These ranges can differ depending on the specific labs per the physician's orders.
*__NPTE:__ >3 mg/L is significant, and you should look for an inflammatory condition.

ERYTHROCYTE SEDIMENTATION RATE (ESR)

ESR measures how fast RBCs fall in a sample of anticoagulated blood. ESR, or sed rate, indicates an acute inflammatory reaction. This rate increases due to rheumatic conditions, HIV, systemic infections, and collagen vascular disease.

NORMAL RANGES	
Males: 0 – 15 mm/hr	Females: 0 – 20 mm/hr

MISCELLANEOUS BIOMARKERS

ALANINE AMINOTRANSFERASE (ALT)

ALT is an enzyme found within liver cells. When damage occurs to these cells, ALT is released into the bloodstream. Conditions/lifestyle choices that cause liver damage include alcoholism, celiac disease, Wilson's disease, liver cirrhosis, hepatitis, and liver cancer.
  NORMAL RANGES: 7-55 units/L

CREATINE KINASE (CK)

This enzyme is found in the heart, brain, skeletal muscles, and other tissues. When a muscle is damaged extensively, creatine kinase is released into the bloodstream. Conditions include rhabdomyolysis, myocardial infarction, strenuous exercise, and certain medications and supplements.
  NORMAL RANGES: 22 to 198 U/L

"STOP ACTING LIKE YOU WEREN'T BORN TO STAND OUT... CLAIM WHAT'S YOURS."

—COACH K

CHAPTER 60

PNEUMONIA

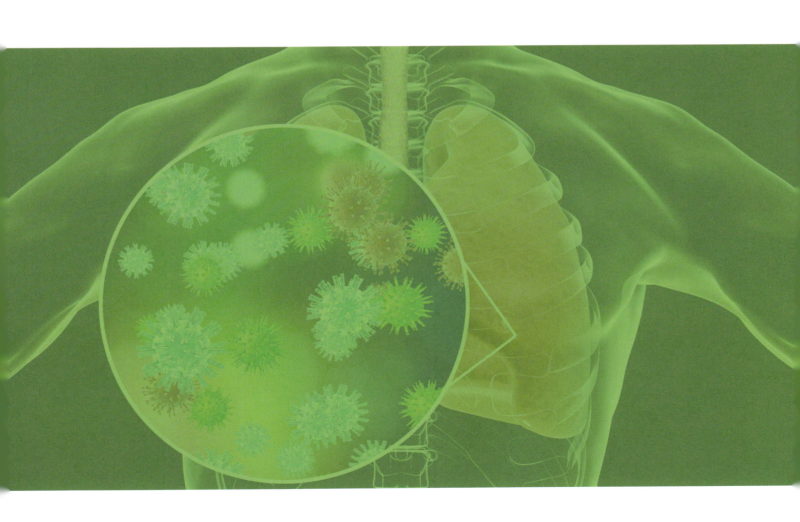

PNEUMONIA[9]

Pneumonia is an inflammatory reaction of the distal airways from inhaling bacteria, viruses, micro-organisms, foreign substances, gastric contents, dust, or chemicals, or as a complication of radiation therapy.

Pneumonia may be in single or multiple lobes, either unilaterally or bilaterally.

4 MAIN TYPES OF PNEUMONIA

- BACTERIAL
- VIRAL
- FUNGAL
- ASPIRATION

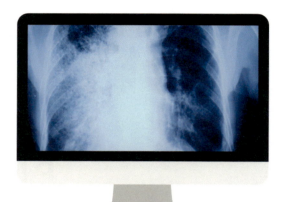

CLINICAL PRESENTATION

OBSERVATION	PALPATION
Tachypnea Fever Fatigue Chest Discomfort	Tachycardia Decreased chest wall expansion on the involved side Dull percussion
AUSCULTATION	**COUGH**
Crackles Rhonchi Bronchial breath sounds over areas of consolidation	Initially dry with progression to productive sputum. Color can vary: yellow, green, rusty, or tan.
PHYSICAL THERAPY MANAGEMENT	
Education Use of Incentive Spirometer Early mobilization Bronchopulmonary Hygiene	

"THE SECRET OF GETTING AHEAD IS GETTING STARTED"

–MARK TWAIN

CHAPTER 61

ACUTE CARE LINES

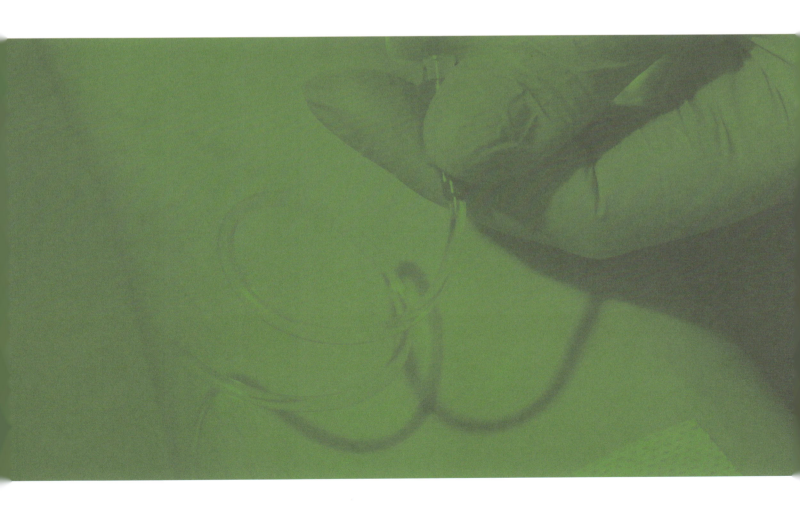

SECTION III

ACUTE CARE LINES

ARTERIAL LINES (A-LINE)

Also known as an art-line or A-line, an arterial line is a thin tube typically inserted into the radial or brachial arteries or the femoral, posterior tibial, or dorsal pedal artery for the lower extremities.

Function:

- Measures arterial blood pressure in real-time
- Obtain samples for arterial blood gas analysis

Commonly used with:

- Critically ill patients
- Hypertensive crisis
- Uncontrolled hypertension
- Post MI

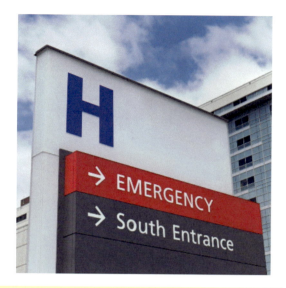

Dr. Rice's Clinical Note
Arterial lines are not typically used for administration of medications. In practice, it is much more common to administer drugs through a venous catheter.

PERIPHERALLY INSERTED CENTRAL CATHETER (PICC)

Also known as the PICC line, a Peripherally Inserted Central Catheter is a long, thin tube inserted into a peripheral vein and advanced to the superior vena cava.

Function:

- Administration of chemotherapy drugs
- Extended antibiotic therapy
- Parenteral Nutrition
- Administration of drugs that should not be injected peripherally.

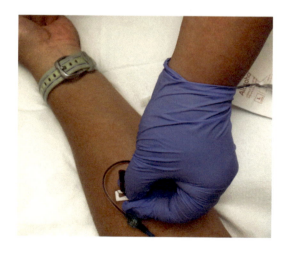

Commonly used with:

- Cancer
- Critically ill patients
- Patients requiring frequent blood draws

> **Dr. Rice's Clinical Note**
> PICC lines can remain in place for days to weeks and deliver proteins, electrolytes, carbohydrates, vitamins, and minerals when a patient cannot absorb nutrients using a feeding tube.

HICKMAN CATHETER (CVC)

Also known as the central venous catheter or central venous line, a Hickman catheter is a clear tube inserted in the jugular vein or other large vein and advanced to the superior vena cava.

Function:

- Deliver chemotherapy
- Withdrawal of blood for analysis
- Monitoring central venous pressure

Commonly used with:

- Cancer
- Sepsis
- Patient requiring frequent blood draws
- Long-term pain medication administration

> **Dr. Rice's Clinical Note**
> Hickman Catheters remain in place for extended periods.
> These are used when the patient receives long-term intravenous drug administration.

SECTION III

SWAN GANZ CATHETER (PAC)[10]

Also known as the pulmonary artery catheter, a Swan Ganz catheter is a long, thin tube with a balloon tip on the end typically inserted into the right side of the heart.

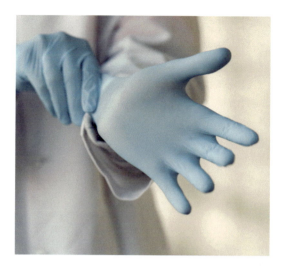

Function:

- Monitor pulmonary artery pressure
- Measure the effectiveness of cardiovascular medications
- Diagnose right heart failure
- Measure right ventricular filling pressure

Commonly used with:

- Heart failure
- Pulmonary Arterial Hypertension
- Heart Function Post-MI
- Cardiomyopathy

"THE PAIN OF DISCIPLINE IS LESS THAN THE PAIN OF REGRET."

–COACH K

CHAPTER 62

PULMONARY MEDICATIONS

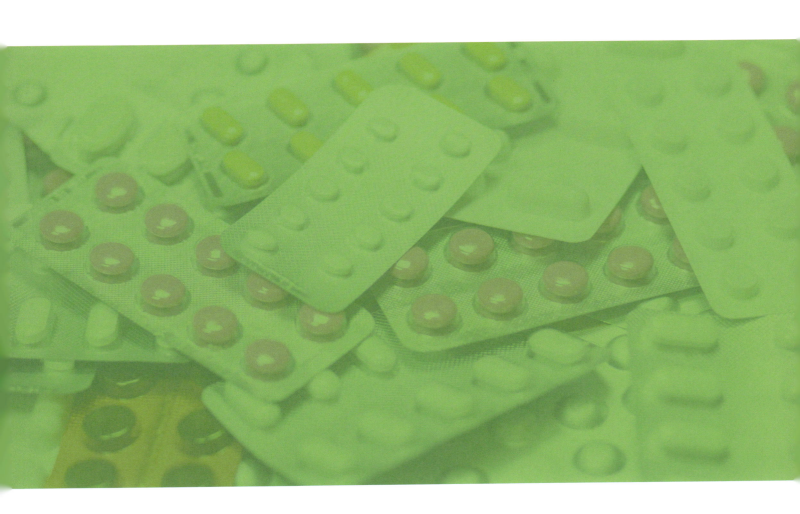

TOP PULMONARY MEDICATIONS

ALBUTEROL (proVENTil or VENTolin)

DRUG CLASS
Bronchodilator: Beta adrenergic agonist

DRUG ACTION
Albuterol is a bronchodilator used to treat reversible obstructive airway conditions.

This medication works by stimulating beta-adrenergic receptors, which relax the smooth muscle tissue around the bronchi.

PRIMARY CONDITIONS TREATED
- Chronic Obstructive Pulmonary Disorder (COPD)
- Asthma
- Bronchospasm

PT-RELATED SIDE EFFECTS
- Tachycardia
- Persistent dry cough
- Dizziness

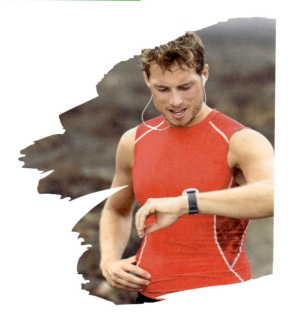

Quick notes:
To quickly remember the function of this medication, look for the word **"VENT"** in the name Ventolin or Proventil. This clue points to the nature of this medication (i.e., it assists with ventilation).

IPRATROPIUM (ATROVENT)

DRUG CLASS
Bronchodilator: Anticholinergic Drug

DRUG ACTION
Ipratropium Bromide is a bronchodilator used to treat reversible obstructive airway conditions.

This medication appears to inhibit vagally mediated reflexes by blocking the action of acetylcholine. Acetylcholine is an essential neurotransmitter for the contraction of smooth muscle around the bronchi.

PRIMARY CONDITIONS TREATED
- Chronic Obstructive Pulmonary Disorder (COPD)
- Bronchospasm
- Bronchitis
- Asthma

PT-RELATED SIDE EFFECTS
- Flu-like symptoms
- Shortness of breath
- Bladder dysfunction

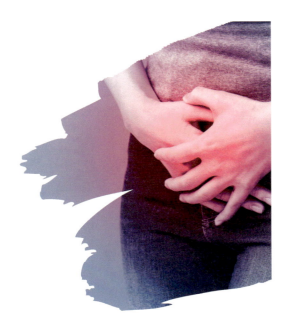

AMINOPHYLLINE/ THEOPHYLLINE (NORPHYL)

DRUG CLASS
Bronchodilator: Xanthine Derivative

DRUG ACTION
Aminophylline is a bronchodilator used to treat wheezing, shortness of breath, and difficulty breathing caused by obstructive lung conditions.

This medication blocks adenosine receptors in the bronchi, thereby relaxing smooth muscle.

PRIMARY CONDITIONS TREATED
- Chronic Obstructive Pulmonary Disorder (COPD)
- Bronchitis
- Asthma

PT-RELATED SIDE EFFECTS
- Angina
- Tremors or seizures
- Dizziness

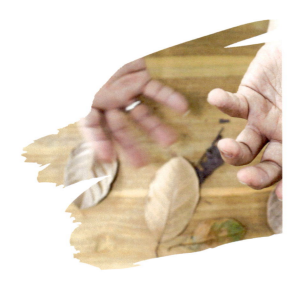

"GO THE EXTRA MILE...IT'S LESS CROWDED THERE."

–COACH K

CHAPTER 63

PULMONARY INTERVENTIONS

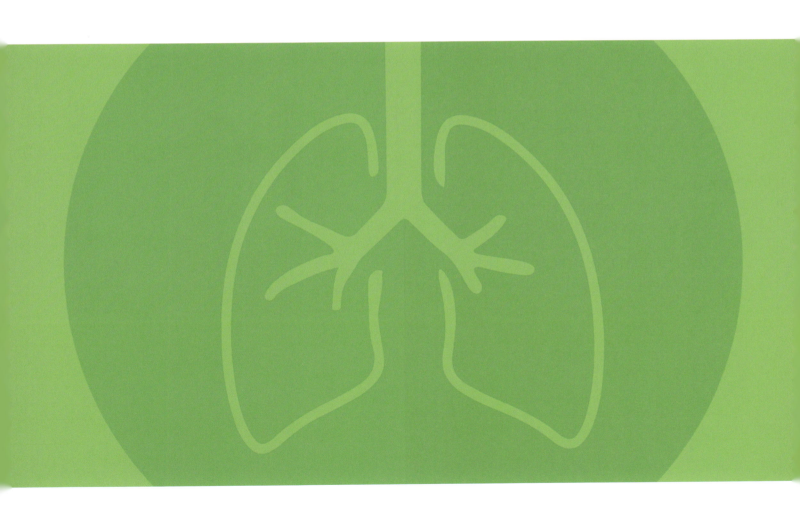

SECTION III

TOP 3 BREATHING TECHNIQUES

DIAPHRAGMATIC BREATHING

WHAT IS IT:
A deep inhalation technique that focuses on activating the diaphragm and improving thoracic expansion. The patient should actively breathe "into their belly" instead of their chest.

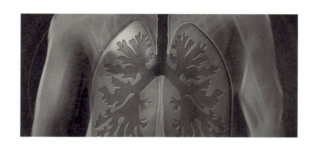

WHO SHOULD GET THIS:
Typically, a patient with a restrictive lung condition. Patients with hypoxemia, tachypnea, atelectasis, anxiety, or excess pulmonary secretions.

WHEN SHOULD I CHOOSE THIS:
To improve O2 sats, resolve atelectasis, decrease anxiety, or mobilize secretions.

PURSED-LIP BREATHING

WHAT IS IT:
A breathing technique comprised of exhaling through tightly pressed (pursed) lips and inhaling through the nose with the mouth closed.

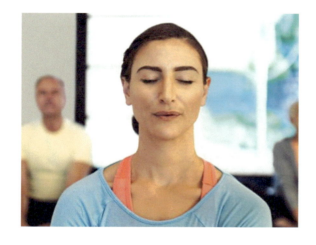

WHO SHOULD GET THIS:
Typically, a patient with an obstructive lung condition who also presents with dyspnea at rest and/or with exertion or wheezing.

WHEN SHOULD I CHOOSE THIS:
When you want to relieve dyspnea, improve activity tolerance, and reduce wheezing.

CHAPTER 63

ACTIVE CYCLE OF BREATHING (ACB)

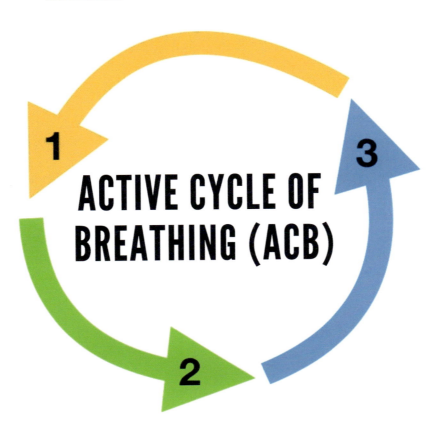

WHAT IS IT:
A sequence of steps that involves relaxing the airways (breathing control), chest expansion, and huffing/coughing.

WHO SHOULD GET THIS:
Typically, a patient who has impaired thoracic expansion and significant lung secretions. The patient must have good cognition, be able to follow commands and be able to clear secretions.

WHEN SHOULD I CHOOSE THIS:
To improve thoracic expansion, oxygenation, and activity tolerance, clear secretions independently, and reduce wheezing.

SECTION III

TOP 3 CLEARANCE DEVICES

MECHANICAL INSUFFLATION/ EXSUFFLATION DEVICE (COUGH ASSIST)

WHAT IS IT:
A cough assist device that stimulates a natural cough by delivering a large volume of air (positive pressure) followed by a sucking force (negative pressure) that pulls the air out of the lungs.

WHO SHOULD GET THIS:
Typically, a severely involved patient with impaired abdominal function who cannot produce an effective cough to clear secretions (e.g., ALS, MS, PD, Muscular Dystrophy, Guillain-Barre, High-Level SCI). This device can be used with patients who have a tracheostomy.

WHEN SHOULD I CHOOSE THIS:
When you want to clear lung secretions, improve oxygenation on pulse oximetry, and reduce wheezing.

ENDOTRACHEAL SUCTIONING

WHAT IS IT:
A procedure that involves mechanical removal of pulmonary secretions from a patient with an artificial airway in place.

WHO SHOULD GET THIS:
Typically, a severely involved patient with a tracheostomy who is on mechanical ventilation (e.g., ALS, Guillain-Barre, High-Level SCI).

A patient with audible lung secretions, desaturation, and/or signs of respiratory distress requiring passive clearance of lung secretions.

WHEN SHOULD I CHOOSE THIS:
To improve oxygenation on pulse oximetry and reduce wheezing.

CHAPTER 63

HIGH-FREQUENCY CHEST WALL OSCILLATION VEST

WHAT IS IT:
An inflatable vest that is attached to an air pulse generator machine that provides a vibration at high frequency.

WHO SHOULD GET THIS:
Typically, a patient with Cystic Fibrosis with mucus plugs and requires mobilization. It can be used in the ALS population as well.

WHEN SHOULD I CHOOSE THIS:
When you want to mobilize solidified mucus in small to large airways, relieve dyspnea, improve activity tolerance and oxygenation, and reduce wheezing.

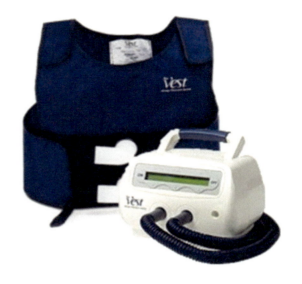

"GO THE EXTRA MILE EVERY SINGLE TIME. WHY? BECAUSE IT'S LESS CROWDED THERE."

–COACH K

CHAPTER 64

RESTRICTIVE AND OBSTRUCTIVE CONDITIONS

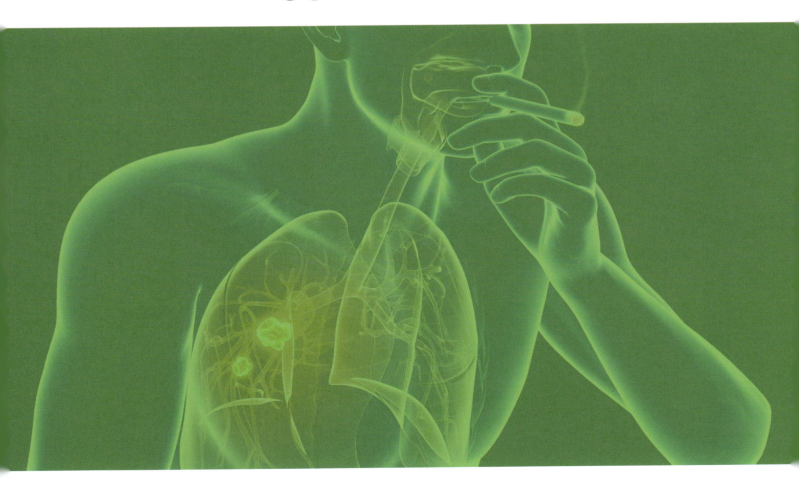

SECTION III

RESTRICTIVE VS OBSTRUCTIVE CONDITIONS

OBSTRUCTIVE CONDITION EXAMPLES	RESTRICTIVE CONDITION EXAMPLES
Asthma Bronchitis Cystic Fibrosis Emphysema	Sarcoidosis Pulmonary Fibrosis Acute Respiratory Distress Syndrome Pneumonia

MEASUREMENT	OBSTRUCTIVE	RESTRICTIVE
TOTAL LUNG CAPACITY (TLC)	NORMAL OR INCREASED	DECREASED
RESIDUAL VOLUME (RV)	NORMAL OR INCREASED	NORMAL OR DECREASED
VITAL CAPACITY (VC)	NORMAL OR DECREASED	DECREASED
FORCED VITAL CAPACITY (FVC)	NORMAL OR DECREASED	NORMAL OR DECREASED
EXPIRATORY RESERVE VOLUME (ERV)	NORMAL OR DECREASED	NORMAL OR DECREASED
FORCED EXPIRATORY VOLUME IN 1 SEC	DECREASED	NORMAL
TIDAL VOLUME (TV)	NORMAL OR INCREASED	NORMAL OR DECREASED
INSPIRATORY CAPACITY (IC)	NORMAL OR DECREASED	NORMAL OR DECREASED
FUNCTIONAL RESIDUAL CAPACITY (FRC)	NORMAL OR INCREASED	NORMAL OR DECREASED

"WHEN YOU FEEL LIKE STOPPING, THINK ABOUT WHY YOU STARTED"

–COACH K

CHAPTER 65

EXERCISE INTENSITY MEASURES

TOP 4 EXERCISE INTENSITY MEASURES[11]

RATE OF PERCEIVED EXERTION (RPE)

A subjective means of measuring exercise intensity that involves asking the patient to rate their level of exertion based on an established numerical system from 6 to 20.

Advantage:
It does not rely on cardiac electrical conductance and is not influenced by electrical conduction abnormalities.

Disadvantage:
Requires learning and understanding of how to use the scale appropriately.

Pathologies/Conditions RPE is used for:
CHF, cardiac transplant, cancer, overweight/obesity, late-stage multiple sclerosis, pregnancy, hypo/hyperthyroidism

HEART RATE (HR)

An objective means of measuring exercise intensity by calculating the number of heartbeats per minute. The exercise intensity can be assessed by comparing the current exercise heart rate to the MaxHR (220-age) or the Karvonen formula.

Advantage:
Quick and objective assessment, readily accessible information, accurate measure of exercise intensity.

Disadvantage:
Unreliable method when cardiac conduction abnormalities or cardiac dysfunction are present.

Pathologies/Conditions HR is used for:
Healthy patients, uncomplicated myocardial infarction, diabetic autonomic neuropathy, chronic kidney disease, hypertension

CHAPTER 65

DYSPNEA INDEX (DI)

A subjective means of measuring symptoms of breathlessness during physical activity that involves asking the patient to rate their level of breathlessness based on an established numerical system from 1 to 10.

Advantage:

It does not rely on objective measures such as respiratory rate during exercise, which can be variable among patients.

Disadvantage:

Requires learning and understanding of how to use the scale appropriately. It is not effective with the cognitively impaired.

Pathologies/Conditions DI is used for:

Chronic obstructive pulmonary disease (COPD)

METABOLIC EQUIVALENTS (METS)

An objective measure of the ratio of the rate at which a person expends energy relative to the mass of that person while performing some specific physical activity compared to a reference.

Advantage:

It does not rely on cardiac electrical conductance and is not influenced by conduction abnormalities.

Disadvantage:

METs are not readily adaptable from one patient to the next because of differences in body weight.

Pathologies/Conditions MET is used for:

Cerebrovascular accident (CVA), Coronary Artery Bypass Graft (CABG), Myocardial Infarction (MI)

CHAPTER 66

ABNORMAL BREATHING PATTERNS

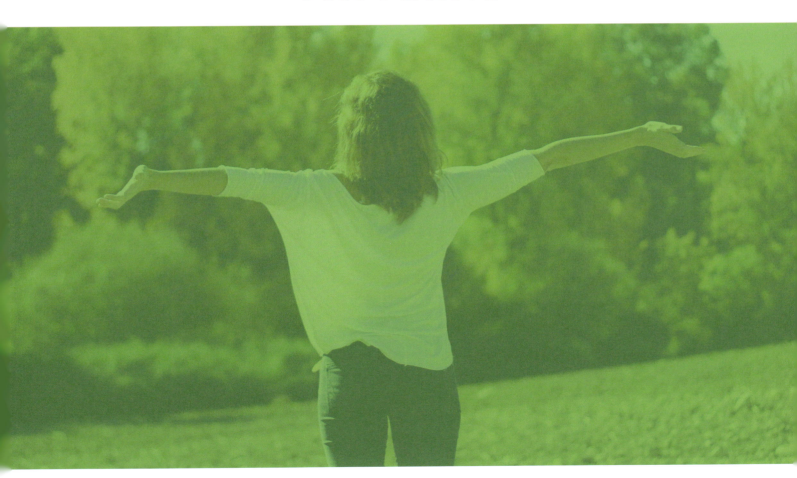

THE FIVE TOP ABNORMAL BREATHING PATTERNS[12]

KUSSMAUL BREATHING

- A deep and labored breathing pattern characterized as hyperventilation caused by metabolic acidosis, particularly Diabetic Ketoacidosis (DKA).
- Kussmaul breathing, also called Kussmaul respirations, starts rapid and shallow, but as acidosis worsens, respirations become deep and labored.
- Kussmaul breathing is a compensatory strategy to increase blood pH by releasing more CO_2.

CHEYNE-STOKES BREATHING

- An abnormal breathing pattern characterized by progressively deeper, and sometimes faster, breathing followed by a gradual decrease in rate resulting in a temporary stop in breathing called apnea.
- A normal cycle lasts from 30 seconds to 2 minutes.
- Cheyne-Stokes breathing, also known as Cheyne-Stokes respirations, is often seen during "end-of-life" transitioning, as well as stroke, traumatic brain injury (TBI), congestive heart failure (CHF), brainstem infarction, and opioid use.

APNEA

- Apnea is the cessation of breathing where there is no movement in the muscles of inspiration.
- Apnea can present in many forms on the NPTE, including obstructive sleep apnea (OSA), the halting of ventilation secondary to airway obstruction.
- Apnea can also be caused by opiate toxicity, neurological disease, or brain/brainstem damage.

APNEUSTIC BREATHING

- Apneustic Breathing is an abnormal breathing pattern characterized by a slow rate, deep gasping inspiration, followed by apnea at full inspiration, and ending with an insufficient release/expiration.
- Apneustic Breathing, or apneusis, is caused by damage to the pons or upper medulla secondary to stroke or trauma.
- Patients with this breathing pattern have poor prognosis.

CHAPTER 66

PARADOXICAL BREATHING

- An abnormal breathing pattern characterized by a reversal of the normal breathing process, whereby the person's chest contracts during inspiration and expands during expiration.
- Paradoxical breathing can be normal in some infants but is considered pathological in children and adults, signifying a severe medical condition.
- Paradoxical breathing is often caused by an injury to the chest, such as a fall, a sports injury, a car accident, or damage to the lungs or rib cage.
- Paradoxical breathing can also be caused by sleep apnea, upper airway blockage, electrolyte imbalance, or neurological problems affecting the diaphragm.

"YOUR BEST TEACHER IS YOUR LAST MISTAKE"

–COACH K

SECTION III REFERENCES

1. https://www.thoracic.org/statements/resources/pfet/sixminute.pdf Hillegass, E. A., & Sadowsky, H. S. (2010). Essentials of cardiopulmonary physical therapy. Philadelphia: Saunders.
2. https://doi.org/10.1161/CIRCULATIONAHA.106.650796Circulation. 2007;116:2191–2202
3. Michlovitz, Susan L. Michlovitz's Modalities for Therapeutic Intervention. 6th Edition. Chapter 5. pgs. 135-148.
4. O'Sullivan, Susan B., Schmitz, Thomas J.Fulk, George D. (©2014) Physical rehabilitation /Philadelphia: F.A. Davis Co.
5. Hillegass, E. A., & Sadowsky, H. S. (1994). Essentials of cardiopulmonary physical therapy. Philadelphia: Saunders.
6. Watchie, J. (2010). Cardiovascular & Pulmonary Physical Therapy: A clinical manual. Philadelphia: W.B. Saunders. pg 278 Table 6-22
7. Wolters Kluwer/Lippincott, Williams & Wilkins. ACSM's Guidelines for Exercise Testing and Prescription. 10th edition.
8. Paz, J. C., & West, M. P. (2002). Acute care handbook for physical therapists. Boston: Butterworth-Heinemann.
9. Paz, J. C., & West, M. P. (2002). Acute care handbook for physical therapists. Boston: Butterworth-Heinemann. Goodman, Catherine C, and Teresa E. K. Snyder. Differential Diagnosis for Physical Therapists: Screening for Referral. St. Louis, Mo: Saunders/Elsevier, 2007.
10. Magee, David J. Orthopedic Physical Assessment. St. Louis, Mo: Saunders Elsevier, 2008.
11. ACSM. American College of Sports Medicine. Guidelines For Exercise Testing and Prescription. 10th edition.
12. Hillegass, E. A., & Sadowsky, H. S. (1994). Essentials of cardiopulmonary physical therapy. Philadelphia: Saunders. Chapter 16 Table 16-4. Pg 547

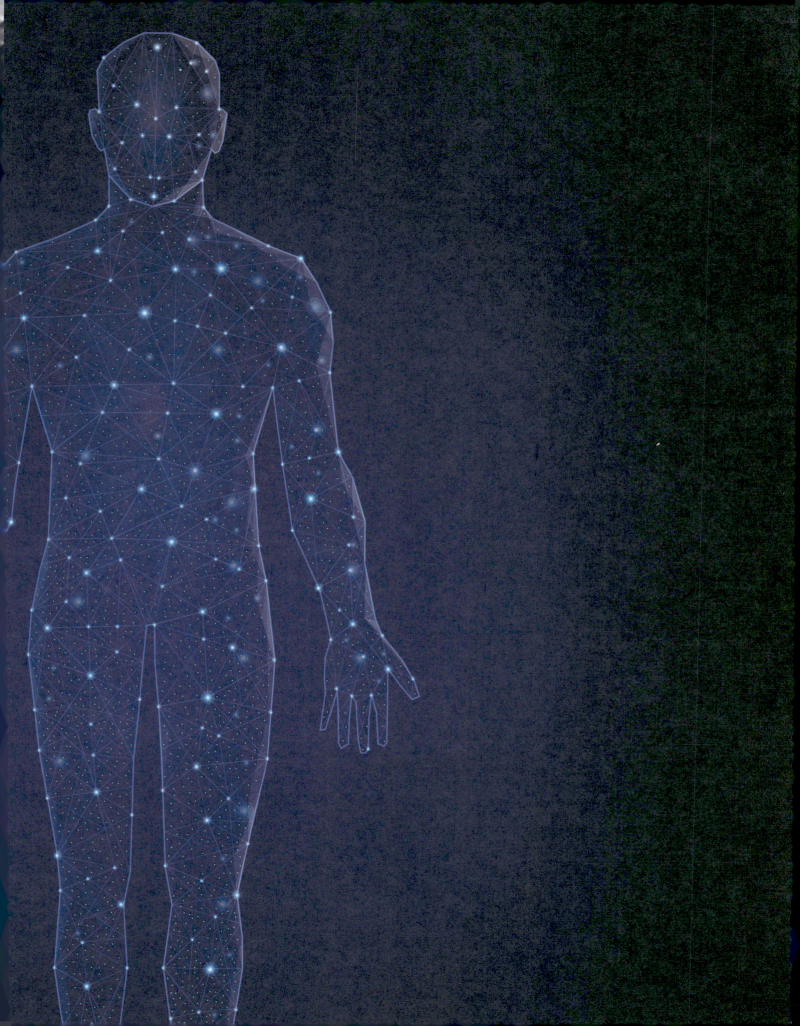

SECTION IV

OTHER SYSTEMS

CHAPTER 67

TYPES OF ULCERS

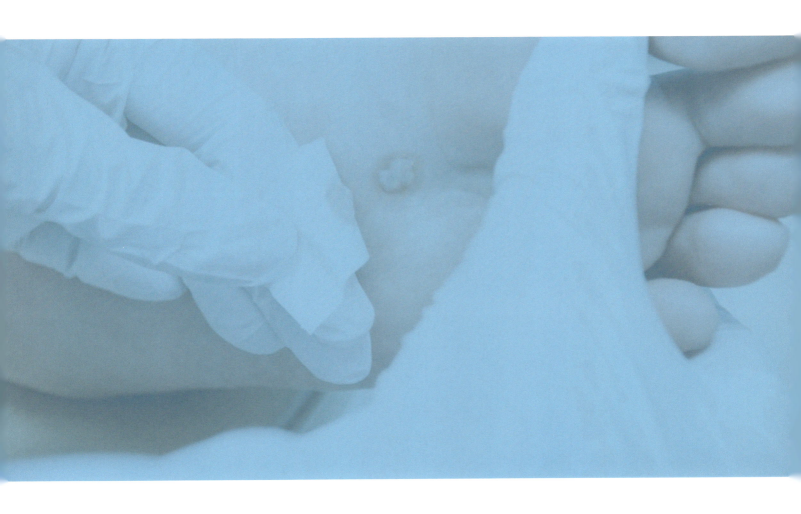

SECTION IV

	COMMON ETIOLOGIES	COMMON LOCATIONS	COMMON MANIFESTATIONS
VENOUS ULCERS	VALVULAR DISEASE VALVULAR INCOMPENTENCE DVT VENOUS INSUFFICIENCY HYPERTENSION PERIPHERAL INCOMPETENCE	MEDIAL ASPECT OF DISTAL 1/3 OF LOWER EXTREMITY MEDIAL MALLEOLUS	NOT SIGNIFICANTLY PAINFUL AND IMPROVES WITH ELEVATION "ACHEY" TYPE OF PAIN NORMAL PULSES CAN BE PALPATED EDEMA HEMOSIDERIN STAINING = DARKENED AREAS OF PIGMENT SHALLOW WITH HEAVY DRAINAGE

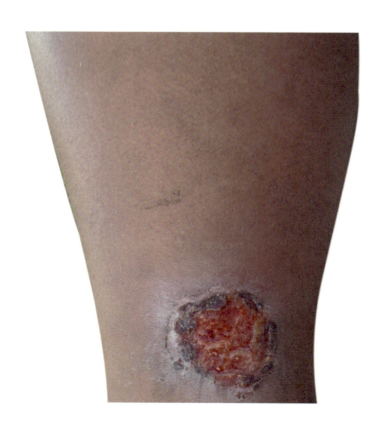

	COMMON ETIOLOGIES	COMMON LOCATIONS	COMMON MANIFESTATIONS
NEUROPATHIC ULCERS	DIABETES MELLITUS ARTERIAL DISEASE (PERIPHERAL NEUROPATHY) REPETITIVE TRAUMA TO AREAS OF POOR SENSATION	THE SAME AREAS AS THE ARTERIAL WOUNDS, INCLUDING THE DORSAL SIDE OF THE FOOT & TOES BONY PROMINENCES LATERAL MALLEOLUS PRESSURE POINTS PLANTAR ASPECT OF FEET, TOES, AND HEELS	"STOCKING GLOVE" DISTRIBUTION SENSORY LOSS NOT PAINFUL DUE TO LACK OF SENSATION TINGLING/ HYPERSENSITIVITY LOSE ABILITY TO DETECT VIBRATION AND LIGHT TOUCH PULSES MAY OR MAY NOT BE ABLE TO BE PALPATED SKIN USUALLY WARM AND DRY LACKS BLOOD FLOW

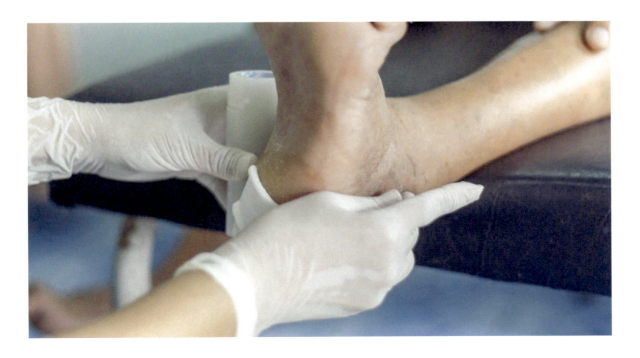

SECTION IV

	COMMON ETIOLOGIES	COMMON LOCATIONS	COMMON MANIFESTATIONS
ARTERIAL ULCERS	ARTERIOSCLEROSIS OBLITERANS ATHEROSCLEROSIS DIABETES MELLITUS CONNECTIVE TISSUE DISEASE VASCULITIS RAYNAUD'S DISEASE	ANYWHERE ALONG THE LOWER EXTREMITY DORSAL SIDE OF THE FOOT DORSAL SIDE OF THE TOES BONY PROMINENCES LATERAL MALLEOLUS	VERY PAINFUL WHEN LEGS ARE ELEVATED PULSES ABSENT OR VERY FAINT PAIN WITH REST PAIN AT NIGHT PAIN RELIEVED WITH DEPENDENCY LOSS OF HAIR & SHINY SKIN PALE SKIN UPON ELEVATION INCREASED SENSITIVITY UPON PALPATION DEEP & TYPICALLY DRY

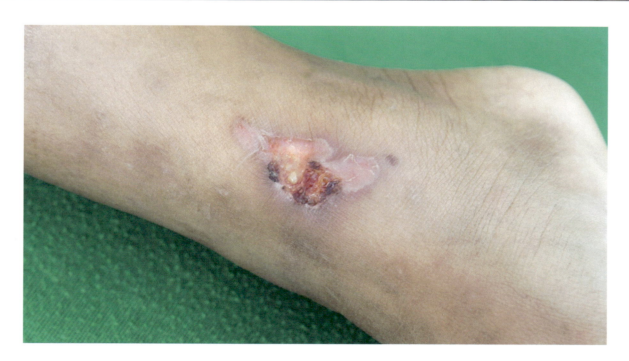

"I KNOW THE STRUGGLE IS TOUGH FOR YOU...KEEP PUSHING."

—COACH K

CHAPTER 68

ABCDE METHOD OF MELANOMA

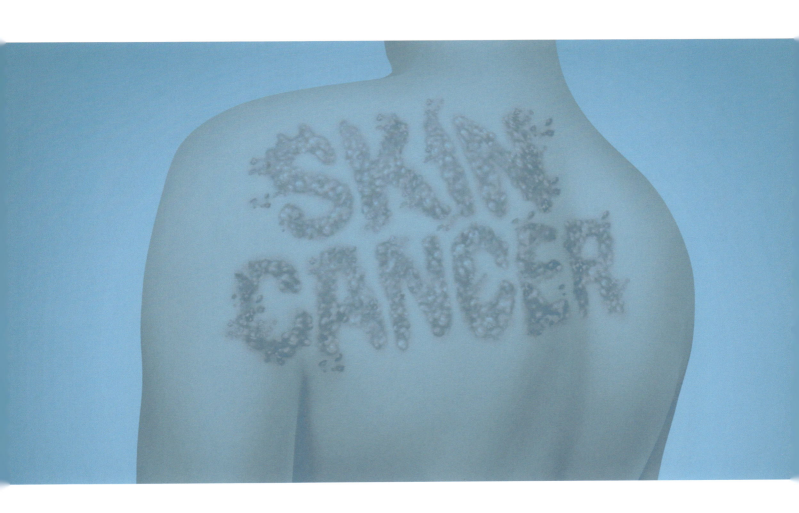

SECTION IV

WHAT IS THE ABCDE METHOD?[1]

The American Cancer Society (ACS) and Skin Care Foundation created the ABCDE method to screen for skin cancer quickly in patients with skin abnormalities.

THE ABCDE METHOD ASSESSES FOR:

Asymmetry

Borders

Color

Diameter

Evolving shape or size

WHEN SHOULD YOU REFER?

A line drawn through the middle of the skin lesion does not produce matching halves.

Borders that are uneven, fuzzy, or have notched or scalloped edges.

Color changes that occur simultaneously with shades of brown, black, tan, or other colors.

Diameter is greater than the width of a pencil eraser (i.e., greater than 5 mm).

Evolving (change), size, shape, color, elevation, or any other new symptoms, such as bleeding, itching, or crusting.

"THERE'S ONLY ONE THING THAT YOU'RE ALWAYS WRONG ABOUT...THE ONE THING THAT YOU'RE TELLING YOURSELF YOU CAN'T DO."

—COACH K

CHAPTER 69

LYMPHEDEMA VS LIPEDEMA

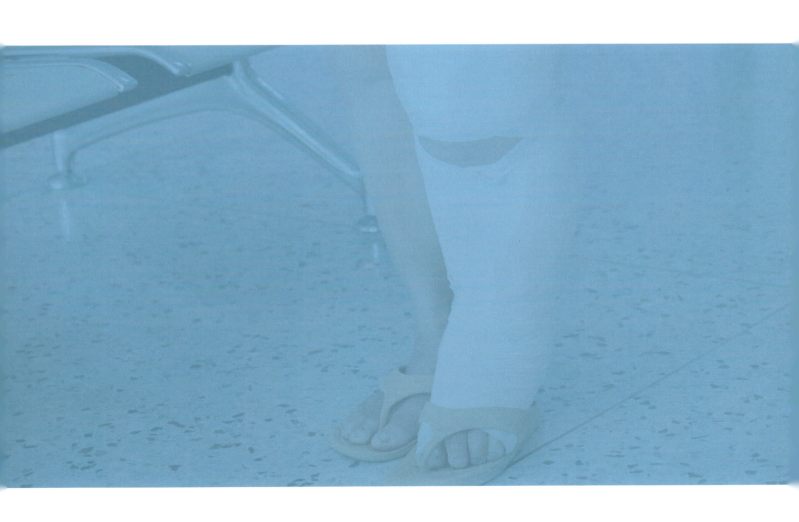

LYMPHEDEMA

A build-up in lymphatic fluid in the body secondary to inadequate removal of lymph fluid by the lymphatic system.

THE COMMON CAUSES OF LYMPHEDEMA

- Lymph node removal
- Obesity
- Radiation treatment
- Infection
- Chronic Venous Insufficiency

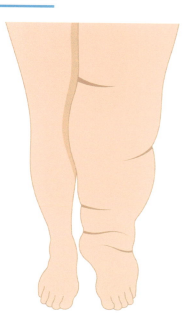

4 STAGES OF LYMPHEDEMA

1. Subclinical stage, swelling is barely noticeable.
2. Reversible swelling with significant pitting edema
3. Irreversible swelling, non-pitting edema, Stemmer's signs
4. Fibrotic skin, large skin folds, permanent skin deformation

LIPEDEMA

- Lipedema is an excessive accumulation of fatty deposits underneath the skin.
- Lipedema is typically found in women's hips, buttocks, and thighs.
- Patients with lipedema have a normally functioning lymphatic system.

DIFFERENTIAL DIAGNOSIS	
LYMPHEDEMA	LIPEDEMA
Affects either gender Mostly unilateral Can be congenital or due to lymphatic system damage Positive Stemmer's Sign (if stage 2 or higher) Swelling can impact the entire extremity.	Female dominant Bilateral & symmetrical Often due to hormonal imbalance Negative Stemmer's Sign Swelling stops at the ankles/wrists.

"BE CAREFUL OF USING THE WORD LATER BECAUSE IT OFTEN BECOMES NEVER..."

–COACH K

CHAPTER 70

BURNS

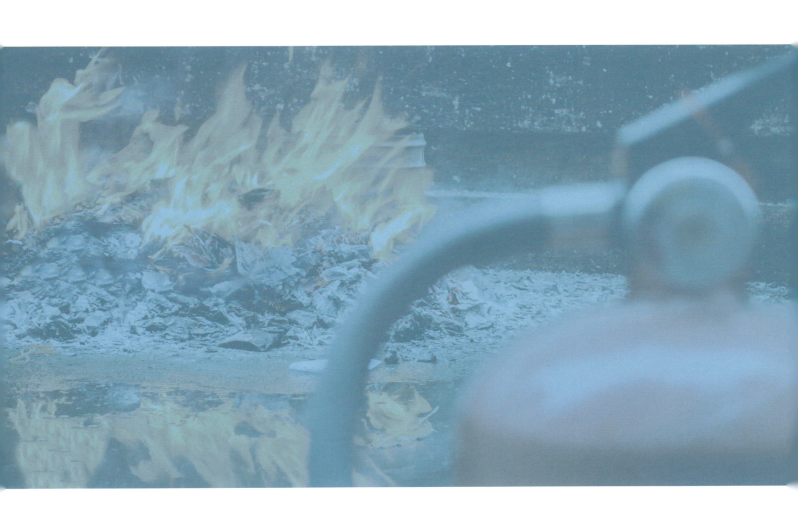

SECTION IV

RULE OF NINES[2]

A commonly used classification method for determining the percentage of body surface area burned in adults and children.

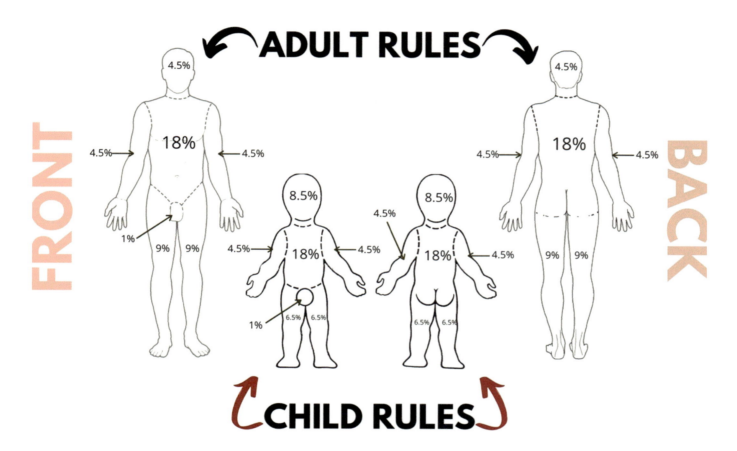

NPTE SPECIAL NOTES:
- The rule of nines classification system has limitations due to the approximation of body surface area.
- Notice the rule of nines does not explicitly address the hands or feet but includes them in the totals for the upper and lower extremities.
- If a question ever asks specifically for the hands, feet, or neck, these areas are approximately 2-3% each (front & back).

"STOP SPENDING TIME COUNTING THE DAYS… MAKE THE DAYS COUNT."

– MUHAMMAD ALI

CHAPTER 71

DIABETES IMPLICATIONS

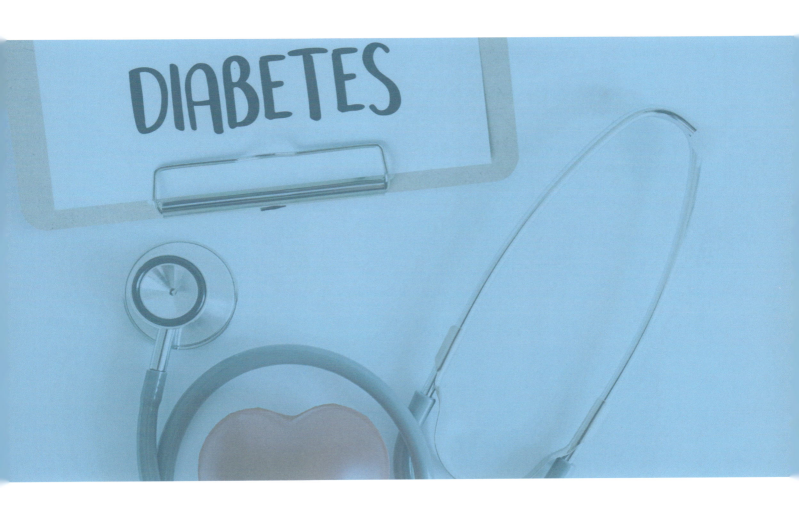

373

DIABETES & EXERCISE

EXERCISE PRINCIPLES

- Safe glucose levels to exercise are between 100 – 250 mg/dl
- Precaution Zone: 250 – 300 mg/dl, no exercise if ketones in urine are present or if >300 mg/dl
- Precaution Zone: 70 – 99 mg/dl; if symptoms are present, hold exercise & administer a 15g carb snack
- Do not exercise during peak insulin times
- Avoid exercise late at night

SIGNS & SYMPTOMS

HYPOGLYCEMIA
- Sweating
- Weakness
- Irritable
- Seizures

HYPERGLYCEMIA
- Lethargic
- Thirsty
- Fruity Breath
- Polyuria

BEFORE EXERCISE

- Monitor blood glucose levels before exercise.
- Drink 16oz of water.
- Eat within 2 hrs of the exercise session (1 hr is optimal)
- Do not inject short-acting insulin in "to be exercised" muscles or sites near active extremities within 1 hour of treatment
- Do not inject insulin in the same location repeatedly. Try to rotate locations often.

DURING EXERCISE

- Follow CDC Exercise Guidelines (i.e., moderate to vigorous aerobic exercise daily, 5x/week, resistance exercise 2-3/week
- Exercise for 40 – 60 minute sessions (if able)
- Eat a readily absorbable snack after every 30 minutes of exercise
- Monitor blood glucose every 30 minutes
- Increase caloric intake 12 to 24 hours after exercise

"I NEVER TOLD YOU THAT THIS PROCESS WOULD BE EASY...I TOLD YOU THAT IT WOULD BE WORTH IT."

—COACH K

CHAPTER 72

PERSONAL PROTECTIVE EQUIPMENT

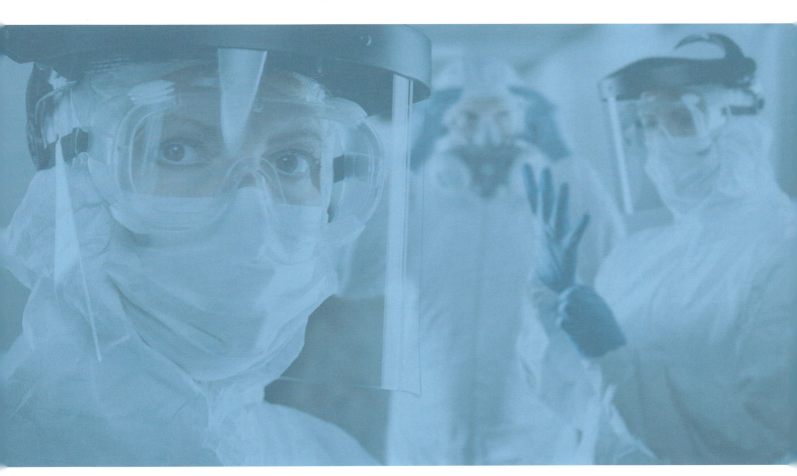

SECTION IV

PERSONAL PROTECTIVE EQUIPMENT (PPE)[3]

DONNING/DOFFING PPE SEQUENCE

Special NPTE Note:
It's recommended that when studying infection control protocol for the exam, CDC guidelines should be used as the gold standard.

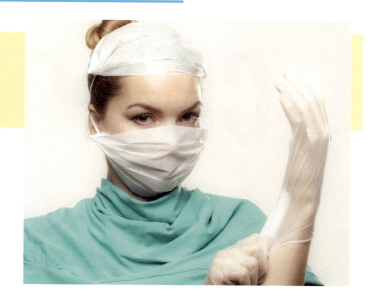

DONNING (PUTTING ON)

- STEP 1: GOWN
- STEP 2: MASK OR RESPIRATOR
- STEP 3: GOGGLES OR FACE SHEILD
- STEP 4: GLOVES

Quick Tip:
Remember to doff the PPE alphabetically when learning the doffing sequence for personal protective equipment.

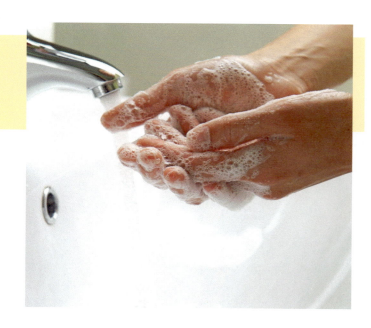

DOFFING (REMOVAL)

- STEP 1: GLOVES
- STEP 2: GOGGLES OR FACE SHEILD
- STEP 3: GOWN
- STEP 4: MASK OR RESPIRATOR
- STEP 5: WASH HANDS

"WHAT WILL BE YOUR LEGACY? WHAT WILL YOU LEAVE BEHIND WHEN YOUR GONE?"

—COACH K

CHAPTER 73

PULSED LAVAGE

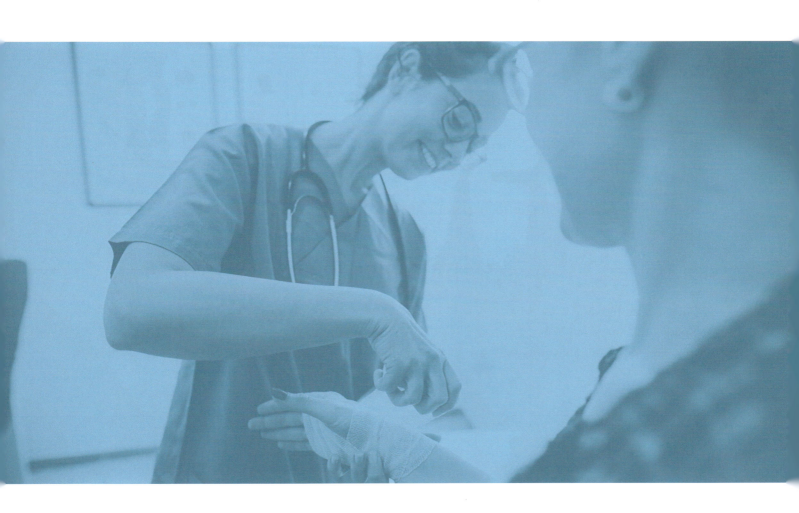

SECTION IV

PULSED LAVAGE[4]

A form of mechanical debridement where pressured water is used inside and around the wound bed to remove loosely adhered necrotic tissue and slough, exudate, and dirt.

PPE NEEDED DURING PULSED LAVAGE

Gown > Gloves > Mask/Face Shield

MAJOR NPTE USES

- Pressure ulcers
- Diabetic foot ulcers
- Venous insufficiency ulcers
- Deep or tunneling wounds
- Infected surgical sites
- Heavily contaminated wounds
- Burns
- Multiple wounds

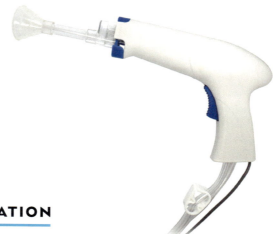

INTENSITY & DURATION

- 4 – 15 psi
- 10 – 15 minutes preferred (up to 20 minutes based on case)

CONTRAINDICATIONS

- Uncontrolled bleeding
- Blood vessels in wound bed
- Granulating wounds are contraindicated unless contaminated, colonized by bacteria, or when non-viable tissue is present

"THE MOST SUCCESSFUL PEOPLE IN LIFE ARE THE ONES WHO CAN ADJUST AND ADAPT TO THEIR CURRENT CIRCUMSTANCES."

—COACH K

CHAPTER 74

TOP NAIL TYPES

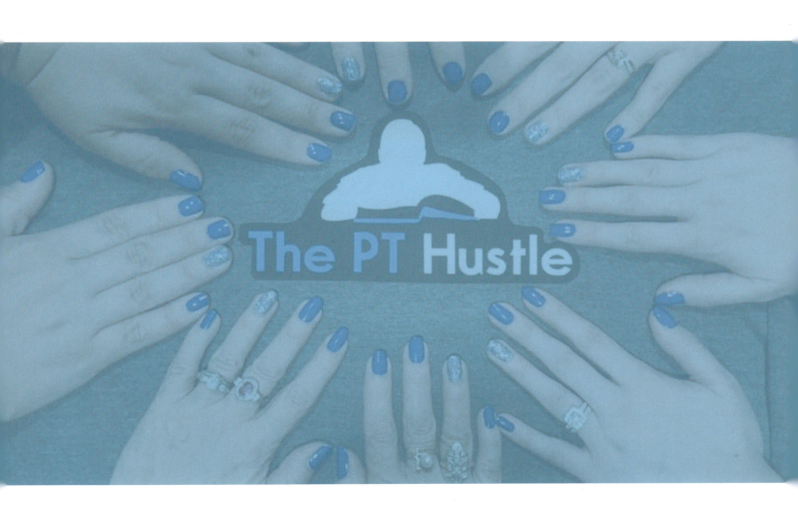

SECTION IV

TOP FOUR NAIL TYPES

NAIL CLUBBING

It is characterized as a bulbous enlargement of the ends of one or more fingers or toes. Several common conditions are associated with clubbing the digits, making it a hot target on the NPTE.

Top Conditions Commonly Associated with Nail Clubbing

    Crohn's or Cardiac disease

    Lung Cancer or a condition that creates hypoxia

    Ulcerative Colitis

    Biliary Cirrhosis

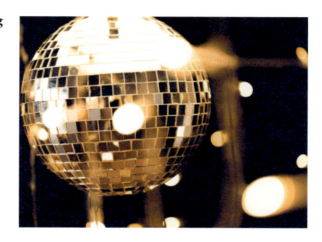

LEUKONYCHIA

This nail abnormality is characterized as a whitening of the nail plate with bands, lines, or white spots throughout.

Top Conditions Commonly Associated with Nail Leukonychia

    Cancer treatment

    Alcoholism

    Myocardial infarction (MI)

    Eating disorders

    Renal failure

    Anxiety

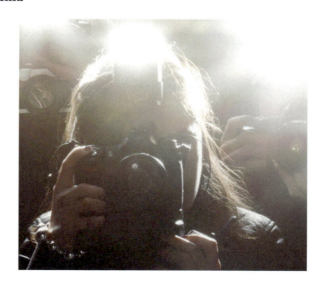

KOILONYCHIA

This condition is also known as "spoon nails" and has the characteristic shape of a spoon. This abnormality is primarily seen in the hands and can be congenital and inherited.

Top Conditions Commonly Associated with Nail Koilonychia

Syphilis

Thyroid dysfunction

Iron-deficiency anemia

Rheumatic fever

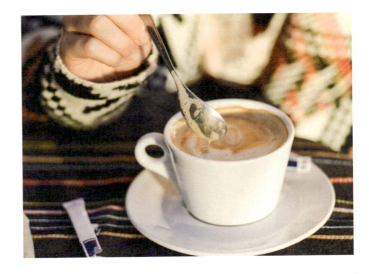

ONYCHOLYSIS

This condition is characterized by a loosening of the nail plate from the distal edge inward. This issue is often seen with trauma, including overzealous manicures, repetitive nail tapping, and nail picking.

Top Conditions Commonly Associated with Nail Onycholysis

Sarcoidosis

Hyperthyroidism / Graves Disease

Obsessive-compulsive disorder (OCD)

Reactive arthritis

Trauma

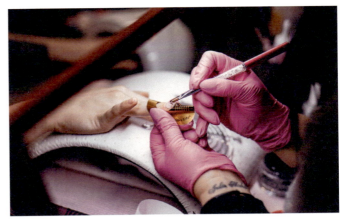

"GREAT THINGS NEVER HAPPEN IN A POSITION OF COMFORT."

—COACH K

CHAPTER 75

CUSHING'S AND ADDISON'S

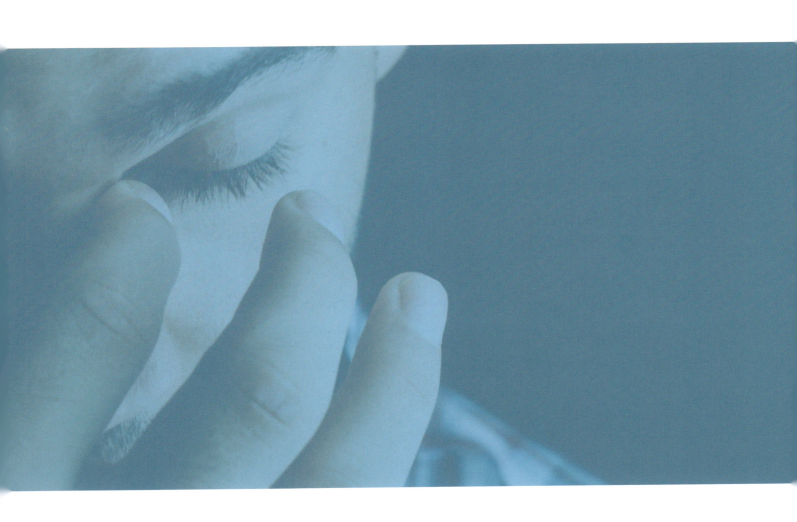

SECTION IV

ADRENAL GLANDS

- Adrenal glands are small triangular endocrine glands that sit superiorly to the kidneys. The adrenal glands have two major components: the adrenal cortex and the adrenal medulla.
- The adrenal cortex secretes two primary hormones, cortisol and aldosterone, which can significantly impact body physiology.

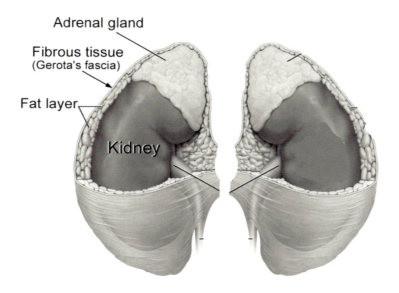

CORTISOL

- Cortisol is a glucocorticoid known as a "stress hormone" that maintains the "fight or flight response" during a crisis.
- Cortisol also regulates blood pressure, reduces inflammation, increases glucose in the bloodstream, regulates the sleep/wake cycle, and boosts energy levels.

ALDOSTERONE

- Aldosterone is a mineralocorticoid hormone essential for sodium (Na) and water reabsorption.
- When secreted by the adrenal glands, aldosterone acts on the kidneys to assist with water and electrolyte regulation.

CHAPTER 75

CUSHING'S SYNDROME

- Also called hypercortisolism, it is a hyperfunctioning of the adrenal cortex leading to excessive secretion of cortisol and aldosterone.
- Excessive amounts of these hormones cause significant changes in the body's chemistry and physiological functioning.
- ***"Cushing's Syndrome is a hyperfunctioning of the adrenal cortex."***

NPTE MNUEMONIC

"M.O.R.E. C.U.S.H."

Moon Face

Osteoporosis

Retention of Water

Elevated BP

Central obesity

Unusual menstruation

Skin striae

Hypernatremia & hyperglycemia

SECTION IV

ADDISON'S DISEASE

- Also called an adrenal insufficiency, this disease is a hypo-functioning of the adrenal cortex leading to inadequate cortisol and aldosterone secretion.
- *"Addison's Disease is a hypo-functioning of the adrenal cortex."*

NPTE MNUEMONIC

"B.R.O.W.N. H.A.N.D.S."

Brown Pigmentation

Reduced Strength

Orthostatic Hypotension

Weight Loss

Neurosis

Hyponatremia

Anorexia

Nausea

Dehydration

Sudden Death

"FAILURE ISN'T A SETBACK... IT'S A SET-UP FOR SOMETHING GREAT THAT'S ABOUT TO HAPPEN."

—COACH K

CHAPTER 76

TOP 7 TOPICAL AGENTS[6]

TOPICAL AGENT	TYPE OF AGENT	INFECTION TREATMENT	NECROSIS TREATMENT	NPTE SPECIAL NOTES	APPLICATION
Silvadene/ Silver Sulfadiazine	Topical Antibiotic/ Antibacterial	Effective against gram-positive, gram-negative, and Pseudomonas infections	Not effective for necrotic tissue	Used for infected wounds and thermal injuries of up to 3rd degree.	Cream can be applied directly to the wound or impregnated into fine mesh gauze.
Sulfamylon/ Mafenide Acetate	Topical Antibiotic/ Antibacterial	Effective against gram-positive, gram-negative, and Pseudomonas infections	This topical agent diffuses easily through eschar, which makes it a great alternative to Silvadene	Used for infected wounds and thermal injuries.	Cream can be applied directly to the wound twice per day. The cream can be left undressed or covered with gauze.
Bacitracin/ Polysporin	Topical Antibiotic/ Antibacterial	Effective against gram-positive organisms	Not effective for necrotic tissue	Used on small/ minor injuries	Ointment is applied directly to the wound and left open.
Furacin/ Nitrofurazone	Topical Antibiotic/ Antibacterial	Effective against gram-positive, gram-negative, and trypanosomiasis	Not effective for necrotic tissue	Used for thermal injuries that are infected. Often used post-skin grafts that develop infection.	Cream is applied directly to the wound or placed on a gauze pad that is then applied to the skin.
Gentamicin/ Geramycin	Topical Antibiotic/ Antibacterial	Effective against gram-positive, gram-negative, Pseudomonas infections	Not effective for necrotic tissue	Used on small/ minor injuries that are infected.	Medicated cream is applied directly to the wound or placed on a gauze pad that is then applied to the skin.

Silver Nitrate	Topical Antiseptic, Germicide, and Astringent	Effective against gram-positive, gram-negative, and Pseudomonas infections	This topical agent cauterizes eschar from non-healing or infected wounds	Used for surface bacteria. This agent will penetrate 1-2mm of eschar and stain black. Can debride dead tissue and cauterize hyper-granulated tissue. This agent can be used to stop bleeding. This agent can burn the patient.	Often applied by using small wooden sticks with a cotton tip applicator.
Collagenase, Accuzyme	Topical Enzymatic Agent	Does not treat infections	This enzymatic agent can selectively debride necrotic tissue	No antibacterial action	Ointment is applied to eschar directly and covered with a moist occlusive dressing. An antimicrobial agent is not required.

"I'M SO GLAD THAT I FAILED 13 STANDARDIZED EXAMS…IT'S TAUGHT ME THAT CONFIDENCE ISN'T SOMETHING YOU'RE BORN WITH. BEING CONFIDENT IS A CHOICE."

–COACH K

CHAPTER 77

HYPOTHYROIDISM

HYPOTHYROIDISM MNEMONIC

"M.O.M.S. U.S.E. S.I.C.D."

SEQUENTIAL INTERMITTENT COMPRESSION DEVICES (SICD)

Pneumatic compression devices are used for swelling and/or preventing blood stagnation in the extremities.

Myxedema
Obesity Or Weight Gain
Memory Loss
Slurred Speech
Unable To Breathe / Dyspnea
Slowed Gi Motility
Excessive Fatigue
Slowed Heart Rate
Increased Blood Pressure
Cold Intolerance
Delayed Deep Tendon Reflexes / Carpal Tunnel

INCREDIBLE OFFER OPPORTUNITY

Are you ready to ace the NPTE and kickstart your career as a Physical Therapist? Join over 20,000 Physical Therapy graduates who have trusted Coach K's NPTE review courses and coaching programs to guide them to success.

Under Coach K's expert guidance, you'll discover the proven formula for answering every type of NPTE question with confidence. No need to spend endless hours studying—Coach K's program is designed to make your prep efficient and effective.

Don't miss out! Limited spots are available, so act fast and scan the QR code below for more information and secure your spot in this all-inclusive program.

Your dream PT career is just one step away!

CHAPTER 78

GENITOURINARY DIFFERENTIAL DIAGNOSIS

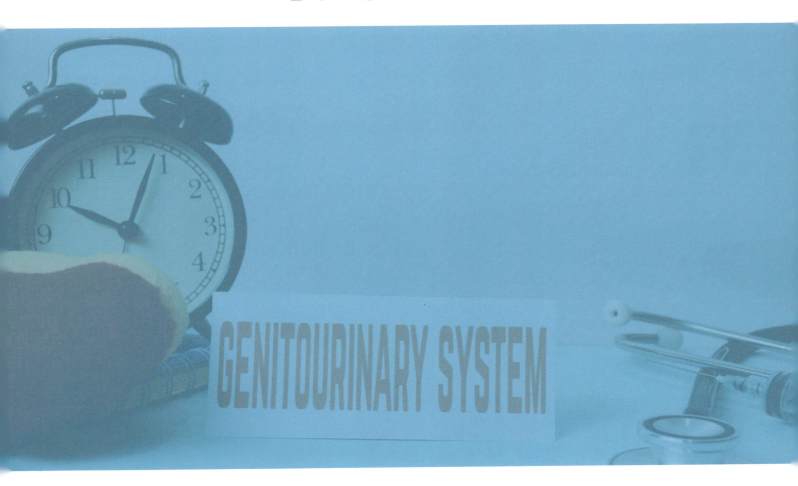

TOP 5 NPTE BUZZ WORDS TO KNOW[7,8,9]

- Urinary frequency - the need to urinate many times during the day
- Urinary urgency - sensation of an urgent need to void
- Hesitancy - trouble initiating or maintaining a urine stream
- Dysuria - pain or discomfort when urinating
- Dyspareunia - painful intercourse
- Nocturia - increased urination at night

PROSTATITIS

- Inflammation of the prostate gland in men typically over the age of 40.
- Inflammation is commonly caused by a bacterial infection.
- Prostatitis can present with the above buzzwords; however, one can expect special signs/symptoms.

Mnemonic

"MY PROSTATE AND BACK IS ON FIRE"

Myalgias

Perineal Pain

Arthralgias

Burning during urination

Fever (moderate to high and sudden)

CHAPTER 78

BENIGN PROSTATIC HYPERPLASIA (BPH)

- A gradual increase in the size of the prostate gland in men, typically over the age of 50.
- Many men live without significant symptoms; however, because the prostate gland is close to the urethra, difficulty with urination, urinary frequency, and incomplete emptying are common.
- Since BPH isn't a systemic pathology, signs/symptoms including fever, chills, and malaise, are uncommon.

When thinking of differentiating signs/symptoms of BPH, think "D.R.I.B."

Dribbling at the end of urination

Really weak stream of urine flow

Incomplete emptying

Bladder pressure (fullness)

PROSTATE CANCER

- A slow-growing form of cancer that occurs in 1/3 of men diagnosed with cancer over the age of 50.
- Prostate cancer is the 2nd leading cause of death in men.
- Prostatic cancer presents similar to a lower urinary tract obstruction (e.g., BPH). This is the case until the cancer metastasizes to the bone.
- Bone is one of the only clinically identifiable regions of metastasis.
- A diet high in animal fat and tobacco use significantly increases the risk of prostatic cancer.
- **"Often asymptomatic and only diagnosed when the man seeks medical assistance because of urinary obstruction or sciatica symptoms."**

Differentiating signs/symptoms include:
- Sudden moderate to high fever (present with prostatitis)
- Sciatica
- Changes in bowel and/or bladder function

"I AM THE NPTE"

−COACH K

CHAPTER 79

VISCERAL PAIN PATTERNS

SECTION IV

TOP 5 MISSED NPTE VISCERAL PAIN PATTERNS & CAUSES[10]

1 THE SPLEEN

Basic Information:
- The spleen is on the left side of the body, in the upper left quadrant, tucked underneath the dome of the diaphragm.
- The spleen plays a significant role in immunologic function by filtering the blood and storing platelets and white blood cells.

Mechanism Of Injury:
- A traumatic accident where the left side of the body is impacted. A motor vehicle accident is the most common cause.

Pain Location & Referral Pain Pattern:
- Pain is in the left upper quadrant and is referred to the left shoulder.

2 THE DIAPHRAGM

Basic Information:
- The diaphragm spans the upper quadrants and is primarily responsible for inspiration.

Mechanism Of Injury:
- Irritation is secondary to pneumonia, local infection, or compression by surrounding organs.

Pain Location & Referral Pain Pattern:
- Stimulation of the peripheral portions of the diaphragm results in sharp pain in the costal margins and sometimes into the lumbar region.
- Stimulation of the central portion results in sharp pain to the upper trapezius and shoulder on the ipsilateral side of the stimulus.

CHAPTER 79

3 LOWER URINARY TRACT

Basic Information:
- The lower urinary tract comprises the bladder, urethra, urinary sphincter, and prostate in men.

Mechanism Of Injury:
- This part of the urinary system removes waste and can be subject to bacterial infection, renal calculi, and other inflammatory conditions.

Pain Location & Referral Pain Pattern:
- Pain in the suprapubic region or diffuse lower back pain (i.e., bladder, urethra)
- Pain in the lower back, pelvis, sacrum, perineum, inner thighs, and testes (i.e., prostate)

4 LARGE INTESTINE

Basic Information:
- The large intestine, also known as the large bowel, is the digestive tract's last part. This part of the digestive system is responsible for the absorption of water.

Mechanism Of Injury:
- Conditions such as diverticulitis (i.e., ballooning of the intestinal wall with subsequent inflammation), Irritable Bowel Syndrome (IBS), and/or Chron's Disease (CD) are significant reasons for damage to the large intestine.

Pain Location & Referral Pain Pattern:
- Pain in the lower mid-abdomen (across either or both quadrants) with referral to the sacrum when the rectum is stimulated by passing gas or defecation.

5 THE HEART

Basic Information:
- The heart is a part of the mediastinum and lies in the chest. The heart is responsible for meeting the O2 demands of the body through pumping blood. The heart can have different referral patterns for males and females.

Mechanism Of Injury:
- Activity-induced myocardial infarction (i.e., permanent damage to the heart wall secondary to ischemia), pericarditis.

Pain Location & Referral Pain Pattern:
- Pain in the substernal/retrosternal region with referred pain to the mid-thoracic area, bilateral jaw, left upper trapezius, left shoulder, and down the medial aspect of the left arm to the 5th digit.
- Women can present with uncharacteristic-like symptoms, including epigastric pain, right shoulder pain, and feelings of indigestion.
- Women can also present with a mix of the normally associated symptoms.

SECTION IV REFERENCES

1. Goodman, C. C., & Snyder, T. E. K. (2007). Differential diagnosis for physical therapists: Screening for referral.
2. O'Sullivan, S. B., & Schmitz, T. J. (2007). Physical rehabilitation. Philadelphia, PA: F.A. Davis.
3. Centers For Disease Control And Prevention, https://www.cdc.gov/hai/pdfs/ppe/PPE-Sequence.pdf
4. Michlovitz, S. L., Bellew, J. W., & Nolan, T. (2012). Modalities for therapeutic intervention. Philadelphia: F.A. Davis Co.
5. Goodman, C. C., & Snyder, T. E. K. (2007). Differential diagnosis for physical therapists: Screening for referral. St. Louis, Mo: Saunders/Elsevier.
6. O'Sullivan, S. B., & Schmitz, T. J. (2007). Physical rehabilitation. Philadelphia, PA: F.A. Davis. Sussman, (2011). Wound Care: A Collaborative Practice Manual for Health Professionals. 4th edition
7. Goodman, C. C., & Snyder, T. E. K. (2000). Differential diagnosis in physical therapy. Philadelphia: Saunders.
8. Goodman, C. C., & Snyder, T. E. K. (2000). Differential diagnosis in physical therapy. Philadelphia: Saunders.
9. Goodman, C. C., & Snyder, T. E. K. (2000). Differential diagnosis in physical therapy. Philadelphia: Saunders.
10. Goodman, C.C. Differential Diagnosis for Physical Therapists. 5th edition. Elsevier. 2013

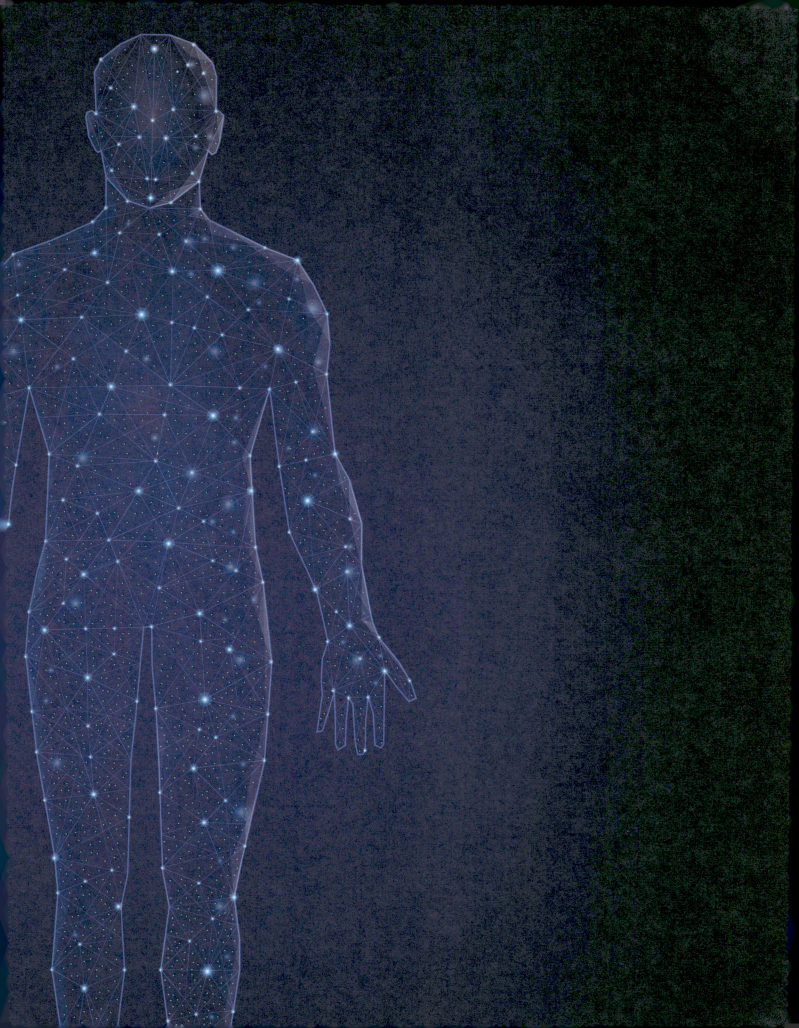

SECTION V

NON-SYSTEMS CHEAT SHEETS

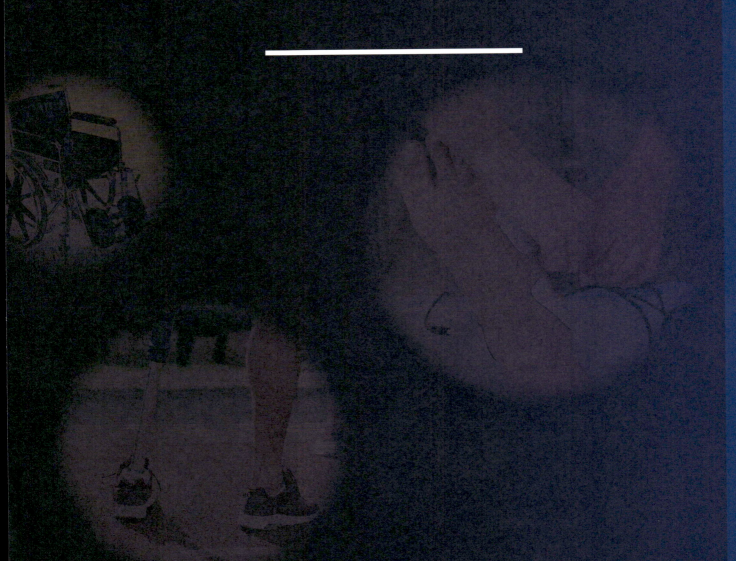

CHAPTER 80

BEHAVIOR CHANGE

TRANS-THEORETICAL MODEL OF CHANGE[1]

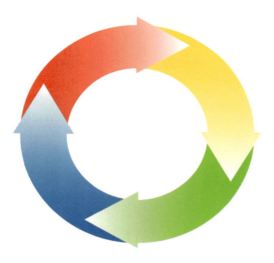

1. PRECONTEMPLATION

The patient is not ready for change, is not engaging in exercise yet, and has no intention of exercising.
Intervention: Provide education and extrinsic rewards

2. CONTEMPLATION STAGE

The patient is not exercising yet but is considering taking action within six months. (e.g., willing to accept information about exercise, attend seminars/workshops to get educated)
Intervention: Provide education, extrinsic rewards, and awareness of the patient's current behavior patterns.

3. PREPARATION STAGE

The patient is not exercising yet but is seriously considering taking action soon, taking the necessary steps to begin acting (e.g., setting up an exercise schedule, buying gym clothes, applying for gym membership)
Intervention: Provide education, extrinsic rewards, and awareness of the patient's current behavior patterns.

4. ACTION STAGE

The patient has been exercising consistently for less than six months.
Intervention: Provide visual feedback to track physical activity and progress over time and opportunities for social influence (i.e., group workouts, accountability partner).

5. MAINTENANCE STAGE

The patient has been exercising consistently for more than six months.
Intervention: Give persistent visual feedback to provide awareness of achieved results, offer greater opportunity for social influence (i.e., group workouts, leading a class, joining a team), problem-solving

CHAPTER 81

INTERPRETING THE BELL CURVE

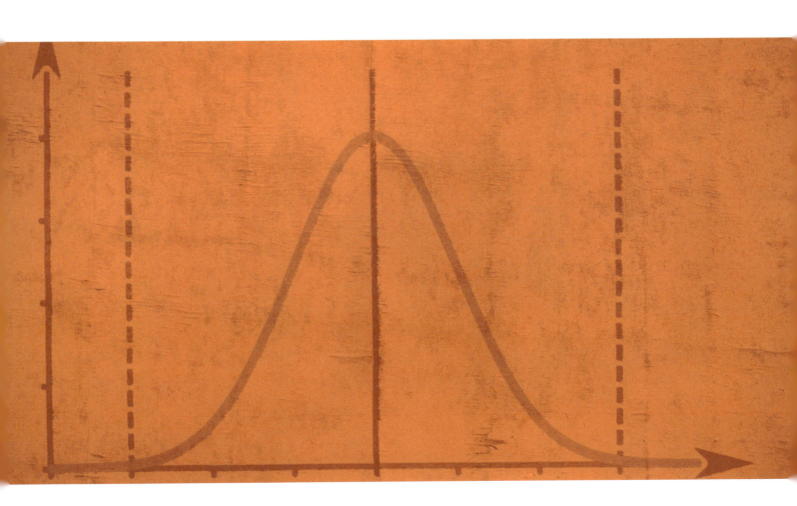

SECTION V

MEASURES OF CENTRAL TENDENCY

- MEAN – The "average" of the data set. Compute this by adding all the numbers in the data set and then dividing by the total amount of numbers.
- MEDIAN – The "middle" value in a list of numbers placed in numerical order.
- MODE – The number or value that occurs "most often" in a data set.

The normally distributed bell curve pictured below is a crucial diagram to know for the NPTE.

Each standard deviation above and below the mean represents a percentage of the total population.

CONSIDER THIS!

When looking at the bell curve (normal distribution) to the right, notice that 50% of the population falls below the mean and 50% above the mean.

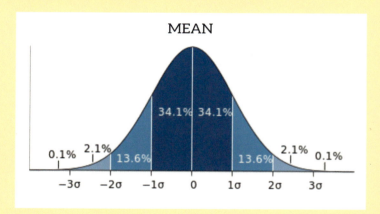

CONCEPT APPLICATION

Suppose a therapist wanted to know what sample percentage fell within two standard deviations below the mean. What would be the answer? (Answer at bottom of page.)

SKEWED DISTRIBUTION BELL CURVE

SKEWNESS – Refers to a distortion or asymmetry in a normally distributed bell curve. If the curve is shifted right or left, the bell curve is called skewed.

LEFT (NEGATIVE) SKEW

- A left (negative) skew is present when most data points fall on the higher side of the scale, and very few fall on the lower side.
- You can always confirm a negative skew when the mean falls below the median value.

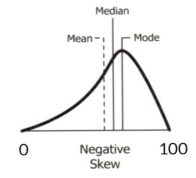

RIGHT (POSITIVE) SKEW

- A right (positive) skew is present when most data points fall on the lower side of the scale, and very few are on the higher side.
- You can always confirm a positive skew when the mean falls above the median value, as seen above.

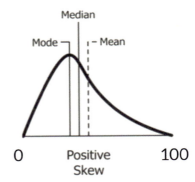

FOOT SIGN

- A quick way to remember your right from left skewed distributions is to use your own two feet!
- Look down at your feet from above and notice that your left foot resembles a left skew while your right foot resembles a right skew!

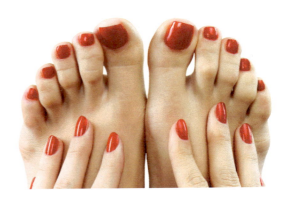

CONCEPT APPLICATION ANSWER: 47.7%

"WELL DONE IS ALWAYS BETTER THAN WELL SAID...DON'T TALK, PROVE IT."

−COACH K

CHAPTER 82

COGNITIVE BEHAVIORAL THERAPY

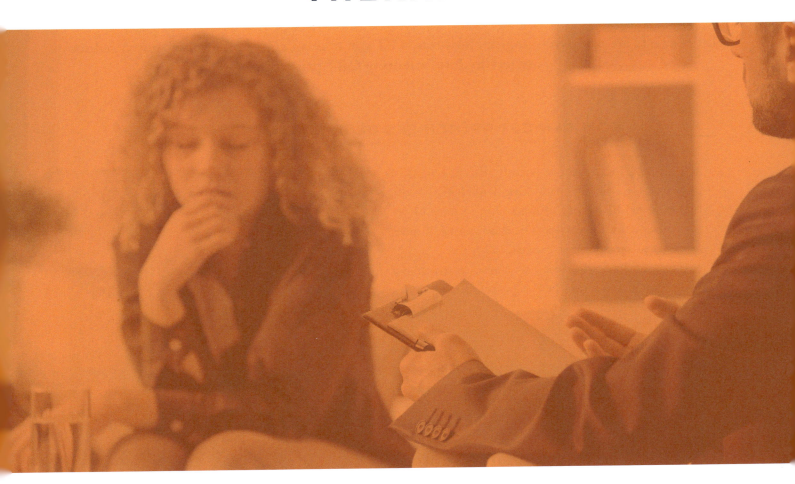

SECTION V

COGNITIVE BEHAVIORAL THERAPY (CBT)[2,3]

Also known as cognitive restructuring, CBT principles help decrease anxiety by changing unhelpful thought patterns and modifying unhealthy behaviors.

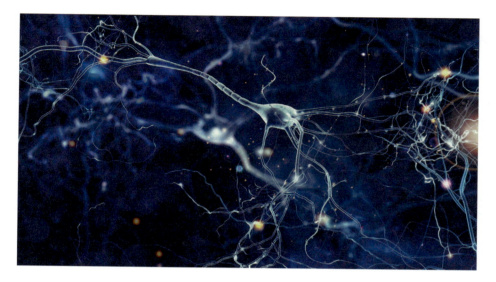

Indeed, PTs are not psychologists; however, a PT can take an active role in helping to reduce anxiety by implementing CBT principles.

HOW CAN CBT PRINCIPLES BE USED ON THE NPTE?

- Helping the patient to identify the first signs of stress (i.e., shaking, nail-biting, fidgeting).
- Helping the patient to determine patterns of occurrence for the anxiety (i.e., daily journal of times of the day and trigger events).
- Encouraging the use of stress management techniques at the first signs of anxiety (e.g., deep breathing)

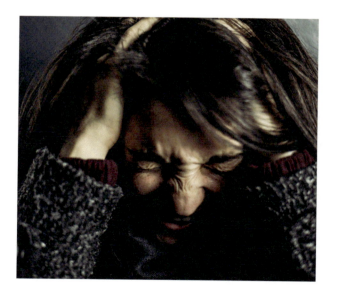

CHAPTER 82

WHEN TO REFER?

- A patient presents with or has a history of panic attacks not previously addressed.
- Generalized anxiety that lasts greater than one week and interferes with the patient's performance in rehabilitation.
- A patient who continues to experience anxiety from phobias despite desensitization therapy and medication.

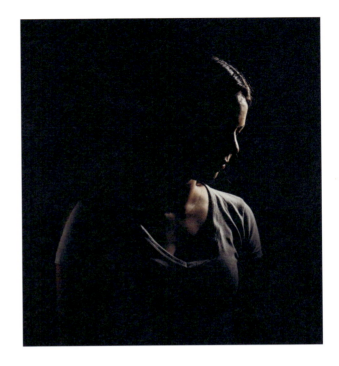

TOP NPTE ANXIETY MEDS

ALPRAZO**LAM** (XANAX)
DIAZE**PAM** (DIASTAT, VALIUM)
LORAZE**PAM** (ATIVAN)

"THE MOST IMPORTANT STORY THAT YOU TELL IS THE ONE THAT YOU TELL YOURSELF"

—COACH K

CHAPTER 83

FUNCTIONAL ELECTRICAL STIMULATION

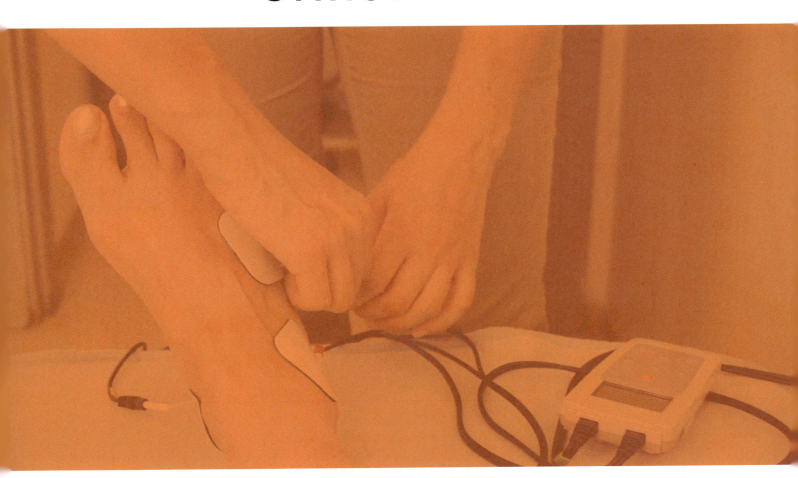

SECTION V

FUNCTIONAL ESTIM (FES)[4]

FES uses NeuroMuscular Electrical Stimulation (NMES) during any functional activity.

COMMON APPLICATIONS

- Reducing shoulder subluxation
- Foot drop during gait
- Impaired hand/finger function
- Exercise to maintain mobility

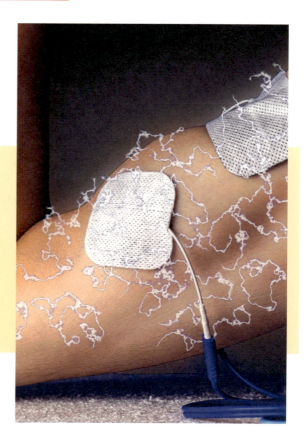

QUICK NPTE NOTES

REDUCING SHOULDER SUBLUXATION
- Symmetrical or asymmetrical biphasic current is the most often utilized waveform.
- Electrodes should be placed over the posterior deltoid and the supraspinatus for optimal results.
- Ramp-up and ramp-down times should be approximately 3 seconds each.

QUICK NPTE NOTES

IMPROVING FOOT DROP DURING GAIT
- Symmetrical or asymmetrical biphasic current is the most often utilized waveform.
- Ramp-up and ramp-down times should be approximately 0-1 seconds each.
- Two electrodes are applied in the proximal anterior tibial region to achieve balanced dorsiflexion, meaning the foot is balanced between inversion and eversion.
- The primary nerve stimulated is the deep peroneal nerve, which innervates the anterior tibialis.
- Stimulation of the peroneal muscle(s) to create a small amount of ankle eversion is acceptable.
- Peroneal stimulation is recommended to avoid an ankle inversion sprain.

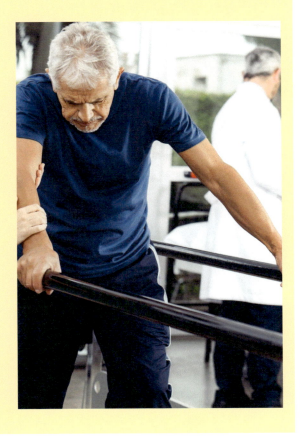

"STAY FOCUSED...DON'T LET A SEASONAL DISTRACTION BECOME A YEAR-LONG DETOUR."

–COACH K

CHAPTER 84

PROSTHETIC K-LEVELS

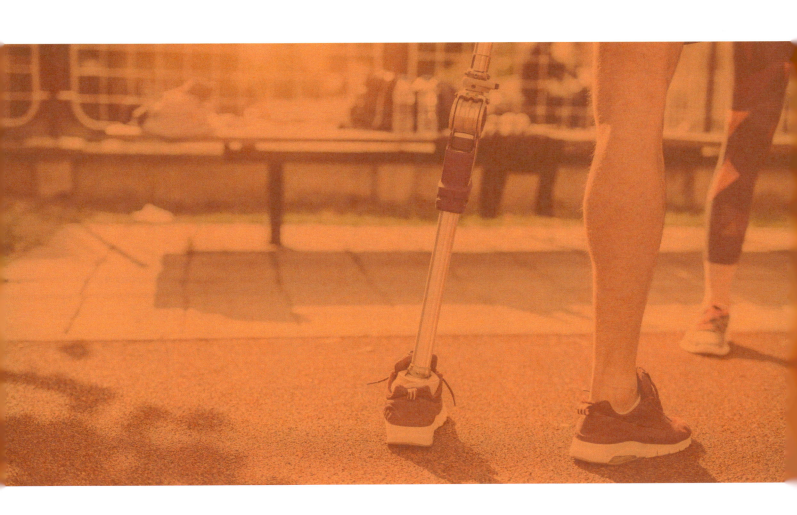

SECTION V

PROSTHETIC POTENTIAL[5]

Not all patients are candidates for a prosthesis, regardless of what the patient desires.

The therapist must consider the patient's:
(1) Level of amputation (i.e., trans-tibial or femoral)
(2) Prior level of function
(3) Cognitive status
(4) Ability to handle the energy demands of the prosthesis
(5) Rehabilitation potential

When determining prosthetic potential, K-levels are a rating system used by Medicare to indicate a person's rehabilitation potential.

K-LEVELS EXPLAINED

K-LEVEL 0: **INABILITY TO AMBULATE OR TRANSFER SAFELY**	• Unable to transfer safely. • Unable to ambulate safely. • Prosthesis does not improve the patient's quality of life (QOL).
K-LEVEL 1: **HOUSEHOLD AMBULATOR**	• Limited & unlimited household ambulator. • Able to use prosthesis for ambulation and transfers. • Level surfaces at a fixed cadence.
K-LEVEL 2: **LIMITED COMMUNITY AMBULATOR**	• Ability or potential for limited ambulation in the community. • Ability or potential to negotiate low-level environmental barriers (stairs, curbs, and uneven terrain).
LEVEL 3: **COMMUNITY AMBULATOR**	• Ability or potential to ambulate within the community using a variable cadence. • Ability or potential to traverse most environmental barriers.
LEVEL 4: **ACTIVE ADULT, ATHLETE, OR CHILD**	• Ability or potential for prosthetic ambulation beyond basic ambulation skills, exhibiting high impact, stress, or energy levels. • Typically, a child, active adult, or athlete.

REMEMBER, K-LEVELS ARE NOT BASED SOLELY ON ABILITY BUT POTENTIAL AS WELL

"IT'S NOT OVER UNTIL YOU SAY IT'S OVER."

–COACH K

CHAPTER 85

PT & PTA RESPONSIBILITIES

TOP 7 MISSED PT-PTA RESPONSIBILITIES ON NPTE

PHYSICAL THERAPIST

1. Physical Therapists are responsible for reporting drug tolerance and/or adverse drug effects to the physician immediately if those effects place the patient at risk for harm.

2. Physical Therapist students are considered an extension of the PT and, when under direct supervision (i.e., line of sight), can perform all functions of the PT.

3. Physical Therapists are responsible for acting in the best interests of every patient and minimizing the risk of patient harm and patient inconvenience.

PHYSICAL THERAPIST ASSISTANT

1. Physical Therapist Assistants shall not determine the appropriate parameters related to the use of electrical modalities.

2. Physical Therapist Assistants shall report suspected abuse involving children or vulnerable adults to the supervising physical therapist AND the appropriate authority.

3. Physical Therapist Assistants shall modify interventions only when it is within the plan of care set up or revised by the PT.

4. Under direct supervision, Physical Therapist Assistants and PTA students can train patients with an assistive device (AD) once the PT has formally assessed the patient and has identified the correct assistive device.

CHAPTER 86

STATISTICAL POWER

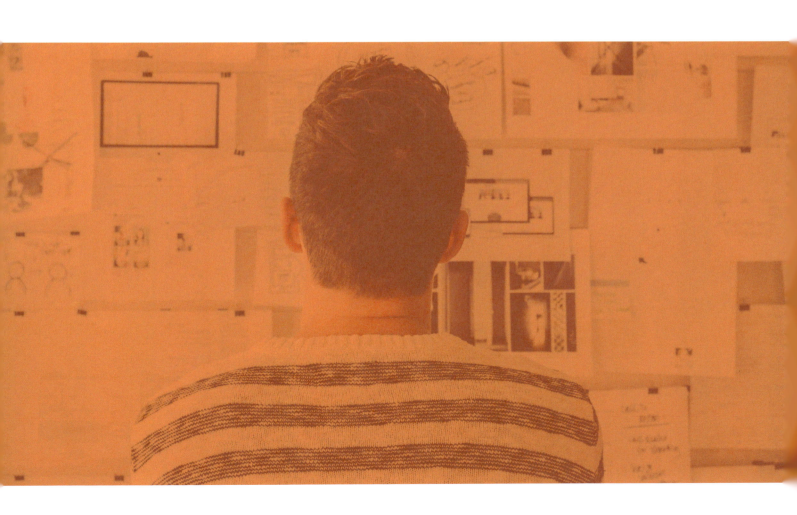

SECTION V

UNDERSTANDING POWER IN RESEARCH[6]

Power is the chance or percentage of a researcher finding a significant result (an effect) in a sample if a significant result exists.

- The power in a study is often set to .80, which is considered acceptable.
- A study with low power has a low chance of finding a significant result when a significant result is present (i.e., type II error).

NPTE TOP 3 POWER INFLUENCERS

1. **Beta value** is the chance of making a type II error and is considered inversely proportional to power.

2. **Variance**, or dispersion, is the degree of difference (variability) amongst a data set. As the variance within groups increases, the power will decrease. Variance is, therefore, inversely proportional to statistical power.

3. **Sample size** is the number of subjects that are a part of the study and is proportional to the power.

"DON'T PROMISE... JUST PROVE"

–COACH K

CHAPTER 87

TENS

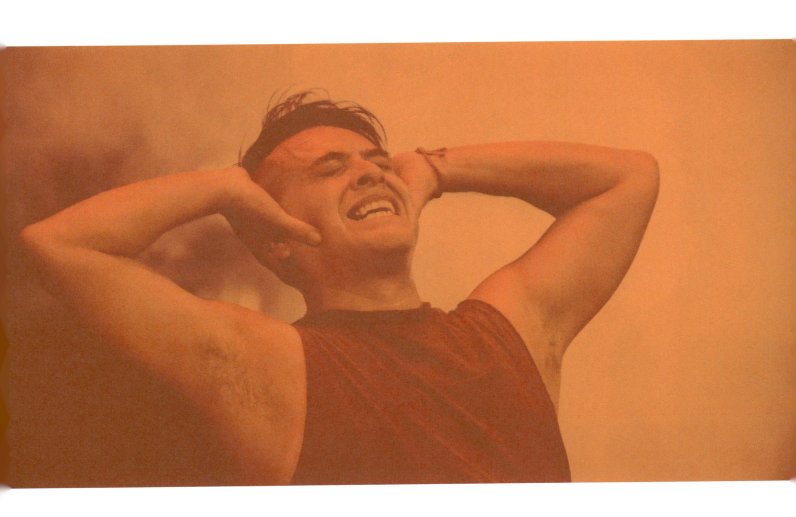

SECTION V

TRANSCUTANEOUS ELECTRICAL NERVE STIMULATION (TENS)[7]

WHAT IS TENS?

The use of low-voltage electrical currents produced by a machine to reduce pain (i.e., analgesia).

NPTE TENS TOP THREE
CONVENTIONAL (TRADITIONAL) HIGH-FREQUENCY TENS
ACUPUNCTURE-LIKE TENS (LOW-RATE TENS)
BRIEF-INTENSE TENS

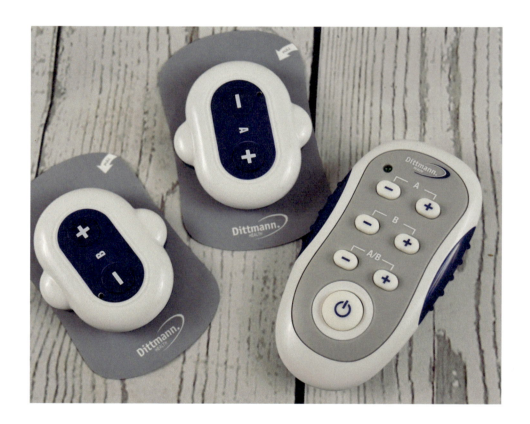

CHAPTER 87

WHAT SETTING SHOULD BE USED FOR ACUTE PAIN?

CONVENTIONAL (TRADITIONAL) HIGH-FREQUENCY TENS

- The most used setting of TENS
- It is considered **sensory only** and does not evoke muscular contractions.
- Conventional TENS stimulates alpha fibers to block pain signals (i.e., gate theory) at the spinal cord.
- This form of TENS can be used for various conditions; however, the effects of this modality are short-lived.
  - *Frequency: 50 - 150 Hertz (Hz) or Pulses Per Second (pps)*
  - *Pulse Duration: 50 - 100 microseconds*
  - *Intensity: Strongest possible without muscular contraction or increased pain.*

WHAT SETTING SHOULD BE USED FOR CHRONIC PAIN?

ACUPUNCTURE-LIKE TENS (LOW-RATE TENS)

- A common form of TENS used for patients who present with persistent pain or are diagnosed with central sensitization.
- This form of TENS is considered noxious and produces controlled pain and muscular contractions.
- Low-rate TENS aims to produce a different but tolerable pain that can release endogenous opiates (i.e., enkephalins) within the body.
- Low-rate TENS produces longer-lasting pain relief but can irritate an acute pathology.
  - *Frequency: Below 10, Usually 1-4 Hertz (Hz) or Pulsed Per Second (pps)*
  - *Pulse Duration: 200+ microseconds*
  - *Intensity: High enough to evoke visible muscular contractions*

WHAT SETTING SHOULD BE USED FOR PROCEDURAL PAIN?

BRIEF-INTENSE TENS

- A common form of TENS used when a patient is undergoing a painful procedure.
- This form of TENS can be used during debridement, dressing changes, or painful manual therapy.
- The purpose of brief-intense TENS is to block pain created by the procedure.
- This is achieved by inducing a new pain that stimulates the release of endogenous opiates through the descending pain inhibition pathway.
  - *Frequency: 100 - 150 Hertz (Hz) or Pulsed Per Second (pps)*
  - *Pulse Duration: 150 - 250 microseconds*
  - *Intensity: Highest tolerable intensity of a brief period (15 minutes or less)*

"CONSIDER IT PURE JOY, MY BROTHERS AND SISTERS, WHENEVER YOU FACE TRIALS OF MANY KINDS"

- JOHN 1:2-4

CHAPTER 88

THE FLAG SYSTEM

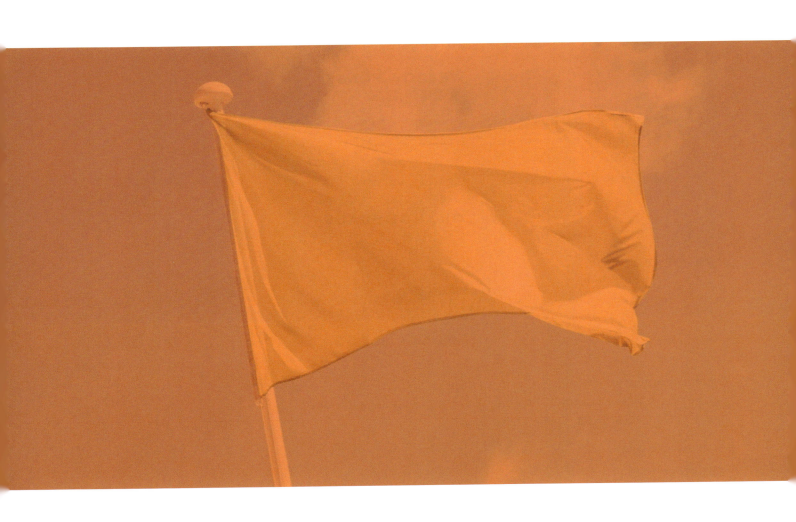

SECTION V

FLAGS IN HEALTHCARE[8]

Clinical Flags & Psychological Flags

These two types of flags are used in healthcare to indicate severe or potentially serious signs or symptoms. These signs or symptoms may require a different action plan or referral to another provider.

RED FLAGS

Signs or symptoms related to serious or potentially serious pathology.
- Cauda Equina Syndrome
- Unremitting Night Pain
- Unexplained Weight Loss

BLUE FLAGS

False perceptions of the work-health relationship.
- Unsupportive work supervisor
- Work likely to cause further injury

YELLOW FLAGS

Beliefs, coping mechanisms, pain behavior & emotional responses to pain/injury.
- Anxiety, fear avoidance behavior
- Faulty beliefs about pain
- Expectations of poor outcome

ORANGE FLAGS

Psychiatric symptoms
- Personality disorder
- Signs of depression

BLACK FLAGS

System or contextual obstacles
- Little ability to modify the workplace to reduce strain on the body.
- Work rules that don't allow light duty.

"YOU DIDN'T COME THIS FAR...TO COME THIS FAR...

—COACH K

CHAPTER 89

THERAPEUTIC ULTRASOUND

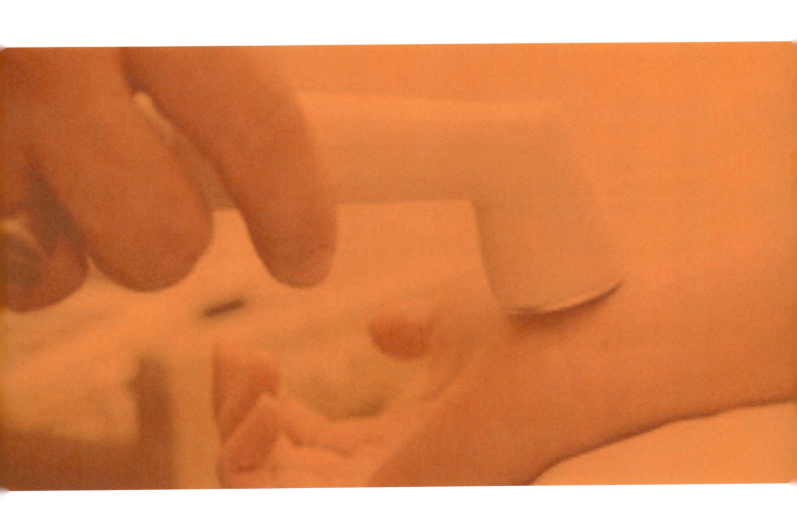

SECTION V

THERAPEUTIC ULTRASOUND

DUTY CYCLE

- This is known as the on-and-off time of the therapeutic ultrasound (US) unit.
- The longer the unit is on and sends sound waves into the skin, the more heat will be produced.
- Duty Cycle is measured in percentages; three percentages are most common in PT.
  - o 20% means on 20% of the time
  - o 50% means on 50% of the time
  - o 100% means on 100% of the time

CLINICAL APPLICATION

100% Duty Cycle

- It is considered a "continuous thermal ultrasound" and should be used to increase blood flow, deform scar tissue, or heat tight contractile units.
- This setting is typically used with chronic conditions.

50% Duty Cycle

- It is considered "pulsed non-thermal ultrasound" and should be used for tissue healing, improving fluid dynamics, and pain modulation.
- This setting is typically used with more acute to subacute conditions.

20% Duty Cycle

- It is also considered a "pulsed non-thermal ultrasound" for improving fluid dynamics and resolving swelling.
- This setting is typically used for acute conditions.

The indications provided here are not exhaustive but give a general sense of when the setting is used in practice.

CHAPTER 89

FREQUENCY

Frequency of the Ultrasound determines the depth, not the intensity.
There are two major frequencies to know for the NPTE:
- 1 MHz and 3.3 MHz
- 1 MHz is considered deep heating and reaches 3-5cm below the skin.
- 3.3 MHz is considered shallow heating and reaches 1-2cm below the skin.

CLINICAL APPLICATION

- Selecting the correct frequency for your ultrasound unit is very important.
- Selecting the wrong frequency often leads to dosing the incorrect tissues with the ultrasound waves.
- When the goal is to provide US waves to deep regions (3-5 cm) below the skin, such as a capsule, deep muscle, or arthritis found in larger joints, a 1 MHz setting should be utilized.
- When the goal is to provide US waves to more shallow regions (1-2 cm) below the skin, such as superficial tendinitis or finger joints, a 3.3 MHz setting should be utilized.

You should consult your Michlovitz text to determine which frequency are best for each pathology.

INTENSITY

This is known as the strength or amplitude of the ultrasonic waves that penetrate the skin.
Ultrasound intensity is measured in w/cm2 and typically ranges from 0.5 – 2.0 w/cm2
- POWER (watts = **w**)
- Effective Radiating Area (**cm2**)
- Intensity = **w/cm2**

SECTION V

CLINICAL APPLICATION

- Ultrasound intensity is often a primary culprit for burning underneath the sound head; therefore, close monitoring and careful intensity prescription are recommended.
- Patients with acute conditions typically receive less intensity, ranging from 0.5 – 1.25 w/cm2.
- Patients with less irritated subacute conditions can withstand intensities between 0.75 – 1.5 w/cm2.
- Patients with chronic conditions requiring higher intensities typically range from 1.5 - 2.0+ w/cm2.

These intensities are general recommendations and may change depending on the case presented.

"YOU WERE TRAINED TO FOLLOW BUT BORN TO LEAD"

—COACH K

CHAPTER 90

TOP 10 NPTE MEDICATIONS HIT LIST

SECTION V

#	GENERIC NAME	BRAND NAME	DRUG CLASS	INDICATIONS	PT-RELATED SIDE EFFECTS
1	Baclofen	Kemstro	CNS Acting Muscle Relaxants	Muscle spasms	Drowsiness, dizziness, weakness
2	Fentanyl	Sublimaze	Opioid Analgesics	Moderate to severe pain	Bradycardia, Respiratory depression, Low BP
3	Aspirin	Ecotrin, Fasprin	NSAIDS	Pain, Fever, Headache, Inflammation	Bloody/Tarry stools, Nausea/vomiting, Peptic ulcers
4	Methylprednisolone	Medrol	Corticosteroids	Inflammation, Severe allergies, Flare-ups of chronic illnesses	Mood changes, Visual changes, Rapid weight gain
5	Methotrexate	Folex, Trexall	DMARDS	Cancer and Autoimmune conditions	Mouth sores, Anemia, Bloody or Tarry stools
6	Furosemide	Lasix	Diuretics	Swelling (edema), CHF, Liver or kidney disease, Hypertension	Tinnitus, Jaundice, Severe pain in upper stomach
7	Metoprolol	Lopressor	Beta-Blockers	Chest pain, Hypertension, CHF, Arrhythmia	Dizziness, Depression, Dry mouth
8	Enalapril	Vasotec	Ace-Inhibitors	Hypertension, CHF	Dry cough, Swelling, Confusion, Tachycardia
9	Diltiazem	Cardizem	Calcium-Channel Blockers	Hypertension, Chest pain, Arrhythmia	Dizziness, Drowsiness, Mood changes, SOB, Swelling
10	Digitalis/Digoxin	Lanoxen/Digox	Cardiac Glycosides	CHF	Bradycardia, Bloody/Tarry stools, Halos

CHAPTER 91

TOP 10 NPTE OUTCOME MEASURES

SECTION V

TOP 10 OUTCOME MEASURES

1. Timed Up & Go (TUG)
2. Fugl-Meyer Motor Recovery Assessment After Stroke
3. Functional Gait Assessment (FGA)
4. Modified Ashworth Scale (MAS)
5. Gross Motor Function Measure (GMFM)
6. Functional Independence Measure (FIM)
7. Barthel Index
8. 6-Minute Walk Test (6MWT)
9. Functional Reach Test & Multidirectional Reach Test
10. BERG Balance Scale (BERG)

HONORABLE MENTIONS

1. Tinetti Balance & Gait Assessment
2. Dynamic Gaze Assessment (DGA)
3. Modified Hoehn & Yahr Staging Scale (H&Y)
4. Dizziness Handicap Inventory (DHI)
5. Dynamic Gait Index (DGI)

INCREDIBLE OFFER OPPORTUNITY

Are you ready to ace the NPTE and kickstart your career as a Physical Therapist? Join over 20,000 Physical Therapy graduates who have trusted Coach K's NPTE review courses and coaching programs to guide them to success.

Under Coach K's expert guidance, you'll discover the proven formula for answering every type of NPTE question with confidence. No need to spend endless hours studying—Coach K's program is designed to make your prep efficient and effective.

Don't miss out! Limited spots are available, so act fast and scan the QR code below for more information and secure your spot in this all-inclusive program.

Your dream PT career is just one step away!

CHAPTER 92

WHEELCHAIRS, RAMPS, & ADA GUIDELINES

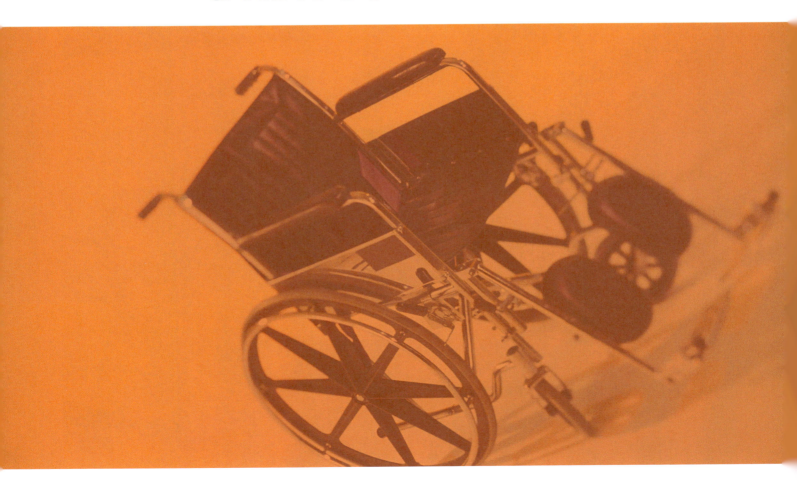

SECTION V

WHEELCHAIR (W/C) QUICK FACTS[9,10]

MINIMUM DOOR WIDTH

- 32 inches

MINIMUM HALLWAY WIDTH (ONE & TWO WHEELCHAIRS)

- One w/c: 36 inches
- Two w/c: 60 inches

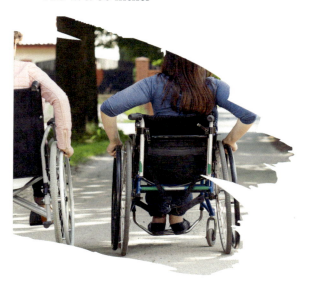
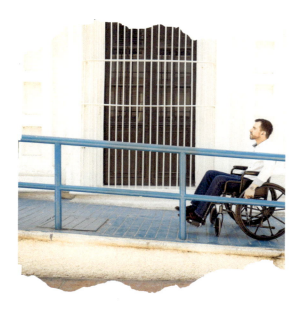

RAMP QUICK FACTS

RAMP SLOPE

- 4.8 degrees or 1:12 ratio

MINIMUM RAMP WIDTH

- 3ft or 36 inches

MAXIMUM RAMP LENGTH (BEFORE LANDING AREA)

- 30ft or 360 inches

RAMP LANDING/REST AREA DIMENSIONS

- 5ft x 5ft

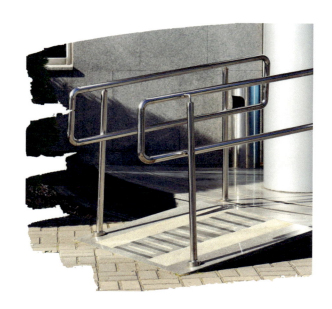

> "THE PAIN OF DISCIPLINE IS LESS THAN THE PAIN OF REGRET."
>
> —COACH K

CHAPTER 93

NPTE ABBREVIATIONS & ACRONYMS

SECTION V

TOP 30 TO KNOW FOR THE NPTE

INTERVENTION/TREATMENT

CONTINUOUS PASSIVE MOTION (CPM)
TRANSCUTANEOUS ELECTRICAL NERVE STIMULATION (TENS)
ISCHEMIC MUSCLE STIMULATION (IMS)
ACTIVE RANGE OF MOTION (AROM)
PASSIVE RANGE OF MOTION (PROM)

MEDICAL PROFESSIONALS

ATHLETIC TRAINER (ATC)
CERTIFIED OCCUPATIONAL THERAPY ASSISTANT (COTA)
LICENSED MASSAGE THERAPIST (LMT)
OSTEOPATHIC MANIPULATIVE TREATMENT (OMT)
PRIMARY CARE PHYSICIAN (PCP)

MEDICAL CONDITIONS

OSTEOARTHRITIS (OA)
OSTEOCHONDRITIS DISSECANS (OCD)
RHEUMATOID ARTHRITIS (RA)
REFLEX SYMPATHETIC DYSTROPHY (RSD)
COMPLEX REGIONAL PAIN SYNDROME (CRPS)

SCALES

AMERICAN SPINAL INJURY ASSOCIATION (ASIA)
DEEP TENDON REFLEXES (DTR)
MODIFIED ASHWORTH SCALE (MAS)
VISUAL ANALOG SCALE (VAS)
MANUAL MUSCLE TESTING (MMT)

CHAPTER 93

MEDICAL TESTS & PROCEDURES

ELECTROMYOGRAPHY (EMG)
FUNCTIONAL ELECTRICAL STIMULATION (FES)
FUNCTIONAL MOVEMENT SCREEN (FMS)
MAGNETIC RESONANCE IMAGING (MRI)
A TYPE OF MRI SCAN THAT SHOWS SOFT TISSUE – T2 WEIGHTED

OTHER

ACTIVITIES OF DAILY LIVING (ADL)
INTERNATIONAL CLASSIFICATION OF FUNCTIONING, DISABILITY, & HEALTH (ICF)
POSTERIOR CRUCIATE LIGAMENT (PCL)
SACROILIAC JOINT (SIJ)
RANGE OF MOTION (ROM)

SECTION V REFERENCES

1. Sull, Eulim & Lim, Youn-kyung. (2018). Designing Health-Promoting Technologies with IoT at Home. 1-6.10.1145/3170427.3188561.
2. O'Sullivan, S. B., & Schmitz, T. J. (2007). Physical rehabilitation. Philadelphia, PA: F.A. Davis.
3. O'Sullivan, S. B., & Schmitz, T. J. (2007). Physical rehabilitation. Philadelphia, PA: F.A. Davis.
4. Michlovitz, S. L., Bellew, J. W., & Nolan, T. (2012). Modalities for therapeutic intervention. Philadelphia: F.A. Davis Co.
5. O'Sullivan, S. B., & Schmitz, T. J. (2007). Physical rehabilitation. Philadelphia, PA: F.A. Davis.
6. Portney, L. G., & Watkins, M. P. (2009). Foundations of clinical research: Applications to practice. Upper Saddle River, N.J: Pearson/Prentice Hall. 7   Reference: Michlovitz, S. L., Bellew, J. W., & Nolan, T. (2012). Modalities for therapeutic intervention. Philadelphia: F.A. Davis Co.
7. Michlovitz, S. L., Bellew, J. W., & Nolan, T. (2012). Modalities for therapeutic intervention. Philadelphia: F.A. Davis Co.
8. Magee, David J. Orthopedic Physical Assessment. St. Louis, Mo: Saunders Elsevier, 2008.
9. https://www.access-board.gov/attachments/article/1350/adaag.pdf
10. https://www.ok.gov/odc/documents/ADA%20Ramp%20-%20ADA%20Compliance%20-%20ADA%20Compliance.pdf

ABOUT THE AUTHOR

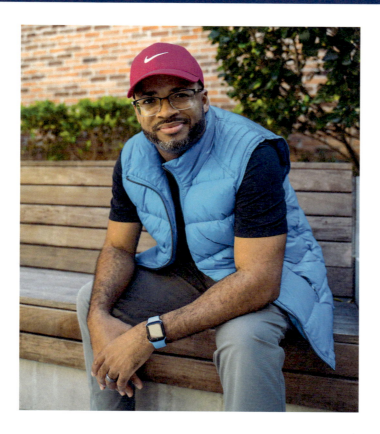

Dr. Kyle Maurice Rice, PT, CMPT, OCS, a distinguished Florida International University alumnus, stands out with an Orthopedic Certified Specialization and Manual Therapy Certification. Scoring a perfect 800 on the NPTE, he's the visionary behind The PT Hustle. For over a decade, Dr. Rice has empowered over 20,000 students to surmount the NPTE, courtesy of his transformative NPTE Cheat Sheets. More than test prep, he's on a mission to eliminate the stigma around standardized test failures, championing students facing test anxieties and learning challenges, and guiding them to thrive in testing scenarios.

ACKNOWLEDGEMENTS

To my wife, Andrea Rice, who has shown me unconditional support,
love, and guidance throughout the creation of PT Hustle and these cheat sheets.
I am eternally grateful and blessed to call you my wife.

To my friend Omar Gonzalez, who helped me make my first book a reality...
thank you for making my dream come true.

FOLLOW US

Please follow us on social media or visit our sites for more information.

Instagram: @thepthustle

Website: www.thepthustle.com

Facebook: www.nptegroup.com

YouTube: www.YouTube.com/thepthustle